BIOTECHNOLOGY FOR SUSTAINABLE AGRICULTURE

Innovative Approaches and Strategies

BIOTECHNOLOGY FOR SUSTAINABLE AGRICULTURE

Innovative Approaches and Strategies

Prakash Kumar Sarangi, PhD
Editor

AAP | APPLE ACADEMIC PRESS

First edition published 2027

Apple Academic Press Inc.
1265 Goldenrod Circle, NE,
Palm Bay, FL 32905 USA

760 Laurentian Drive, Unit 19,
Burlington, ON L7N 0A4, Canada

CRC Press
2385 NW Executive Center Drive,
Suite 320, Boca Raton FL 33431

4 Park Square, Milton Park,
Abingdon, Oxon, OX14 4RN UK

Library and Archives Canada Cataloguing in Publication

Title: Biotechnology for sustainable agriculture : innovative approaches and strategies / Prakash Kumar Sarangi, PhD, editor.
Other titles: Biotechnology for sustainable agriculture (Palm Bay, Fla.)
Names: Sarangi, Prakash Kumar, editor
Description: First edition. | Includes bibliographical references and index.
Identifiers: Canadiana (print) 20260207292 | Canadiana (ebook) 20260207322 | ISBN 9781779642981 (hardcover) | ISBN 9781779642998 (ebook)
Subjects: LCSH: Sustainable agriculture. | LCSH: Agricultural biotechnology.
Classification: LCC S494.5.S86 B56 2026 | DDC 630.2/086—dc23

Library of Congress Cataloging-in-Publication Data

CIP data on file with US Library of Congress

ISBN: 978-1-77964-298-1 (hbk)
ISBN: 978-1-77964-299-8 (ebk)

DOI: 10.1201/9781779642998

About the Editor

Prakash Kumar Sarangi, PhD
Scientist (Microbiology), College of Agriculture, Central Agricultural University, Imphal, India

Prakash Kumar Sarangi, PhD, is a Scientist with specialization in microbiology at the Central Agricultural University, Imphal, India. He holds a PhD in Microbial Biotechnology from Ravenshaw University, India, and an MTech degree from the Department of Agriculture and Food Engineering, Indian Institute of Technology Kharagpur, India. Dr. Sarangi's research focuses on bioprocess engineering, biochemicals, biomaterials, and sustainable development. His expertise lies in the bioconversion of biomass into biofuels, biochemicals, and nutraceuticals, as well as environmental waste remediation. He has taken leading roles as the principal investigator in various R&D projects on biomass conversion and microbial biodegradation into value-added products. He has more than 15 years of teaching and research experience in biochemical engineering, microbial biotechnology, downstream processing, food microbiology, and molecular biology. He serves as an editorial board member for several international journals, including *PLOS ONE, 3 Biotech,* and *Biofuels, Bioproducts and Biorefining.* He is also a guest editor for the *Journal of Biomass Conversion and Biorefinery, Chemical Engineering and Technology, and Biofuels, Bioproducts and Biorefining.* He has published more than 130 research articles in peer-reviewed journals and contributed to over 75 book chapters. He has presented his work at numerous national and international conferences. Dr. Sarangi is affiliated with many scientific societies, including as a fellow member of the Society for Applied Biotechnology and a life member of the Biotech Research Society of India, Society for Biotechnologists of India, Association of Microbiologists of India, Indian Science Congress Association, Forum of Scientists, Engineers & Technologists, and the International Association of Academicians and Researchers. He has also authored several books in the field of biomass conversion and value addition.

Contents

Contributors

Licon Kumar Acharya
ICAR–National Research Center for Integrated Pest Management, Pusa Campus, New Delhi, Delhi, India

Tusi Chakma
College of Agriculture, Central Agricultural University, Imphal, Manipur, India

Kota Chakrapani
College of Agriculture, Central Agricultural University, Imphal, Manipur, India

Subhash Chander
ICAR–National Research Center for Integrated Pest Management, Pusa Campus, New Delhi, Delhi, India

W. Tampakleima Chanu
College of Agriculture, Central Agricultural University, Imphal, Manipur, India

Ahmad Gazali
Department of Biotechnology, School of Life Sciences, Mahatma Gandhi Central University, Motihari, Bihar, India

Rahul Gupta
Amity Institute of Biotechnology, Amity University Uttar Pradesh, Lucknow Campus, Lucknow, Uttar Pradesh, India

M. K. Khokhar
ICAR–National Research Center for Integrated Pest Management, Pusa Campus, New Delhi, Delhi, India

Prabh Narayan Meena
ICAR–National Research Center for Integrated Pest Management, Pusa Campus, New Delhi, Delhi, India

Priti Pal
Amity Institute of Biotechnology, Amity University Uttar Pradesh, Lucknow Campus, Lucknow, India

Brijesh Pandey
Department of Biotechnology, School of Life Sciences, Mahatma Gandhi Central University, Motihari, Bihar, India

Ashna Parveen
Department of Biotechnology & Microbiology, Meerut Institute of Engineering and Technology, Baghpat Road Bypass Crossing, Meerut, India

Anand Prakash
Department of Biotechnology, School of Life Sciences, Mahatma Gandhi Central University, Motihari, Bihar, India

Om Prakash
Department of Biotechnology, School of Life Sciences, Mahatma Gandhi Central University, Motihari, Bihar, India

Devaramane Raghavendra
ICAR–National Research Center for Integrated Pest Management, Pusa Campus, New Delhi, Delhi, India

Uttam Kumar Sahoo
Department of Forestry, Mizoram University, Aizawl, Mizoram, India

Prakash Kumar Sarangi
College of Agriculture, Central Agricultural University, Imphal, Manipur, India

Akhilesh Kumar Singh
Department of Biotechnology, School of Life Sciences, Mahatma Gandhi Central University, Motihari, Bihar, India

Maharudra Pratap Singh
Department of Biotechnology, School of Life Sciences, Mahatma Gandhi Central University, Motihari, Bihar, India

Rishi Kumar Singh
School of Biosciences, IMS Institute, University Courses Campus, Ghaziabad, Uttar Pradesh, India

Bireswar Sinha
Department of Plant Pathology, School of Agricultural Sciences, Nagaland University, Medziphema, Nagaland, India

Bijeeta Thangjam
College of Agriculture, Central Agricultural University, Imphal, Manipur, India

Abbreviations

ACC	aminocyclopropane-1-carboxylate
AI	artificial intelligence
AM	arbuscular mycorrhizae
BBTV	banana bunchy top virus
BNF	biological nitrogen fixation
BV	budded virion
CFU	colony-forming unit
EPA	Environmental Protection Agency
EPF	entomopathogenic fungi
EPN	entomopathogenic nematode
FAO	Food and Agriculture Organization
GA	gibberellic acid
GMO	genetically modified organism
HR	hypersensitive reaction
IAA	indole acetic acid
IJ	infective-stage juvenile
IPM	integrated pest management
ISFM	integrated soil fertility management
ISR	induces systemic resistance
LE	larval equivalent
LPS	lipopolysaccharides
MIR	microbial induced resistance
NPV	nuclear polyhedrosis virus
OBs	occlusion bodies
ODV	occluded body derived virion
PAL	phenylalanine ammonia-lyase
PCR	polymerase chain reaction
PGPF	plant growth-promoting fungi
PRP	pathogenesis-related proteins
PSB	phosphate-solubilizing bacteria
PSM	phosphate solubilizing microorganism
ROS	reactive oxygen species
SAR	systemic acquired resistance
SFE	supercritical fluid extraction
SOD	superoxide dismutase
TCP	tricalcium phosphate

TMV	tobacco mosaic virus
TNV	tobacco necrosis virus
UAV	unmanned aerial vehicle
VOC	volatile organic compound

Preface

In an era where global challenges like climate change, resource scarcity, and population growth are shaping the future of food production, the concept of sustainable agriculture has emerged as a powerful solution. Sustainable agriculture is not only about growing food but also about cultivating systems that respect ecological balance, preserve resources, and ensure social and economic well-being for future generations. It encompasses a range of practices—from organic farming and permaculture to precision agriculture—that seek to harmonize human needs with the Earth's finite resources.

The increasing global population compels academicians and researchers to develop sustainable solutions for the future of agriculture. Microbial resources can play a key role in achieving a clean and green environment on the one hand and advancing sustainable agriculture on the other. Microorganisms are among the most valuable natural resources, and their contributions are beyond practical calculation. Microbial communities can offer valuable insights for studying both applied and fundamental environmental processes. Maintaining diverse and functional microbial communities is crucial for sustainable ecosystems. This can be achieved through the engineering of soil, plant–microbe interactions, and crop production systems.

This book explores the principles and practices of sustainable agriculture and the transformative role it plays in addressing the critical issues facing our world today. Readers will journey through diverse farming approaches that emphasize soil health, biodiversity, water conservation, and resilience to climate variability. Moreover, the book delves into the socio-economic dimensions of sustainable agriculture, highlighting how these practices can empower communities, improve food security, and contribute to rural development.

The editor extends appreciation to the contributing authors for their valuable input in shaping the content of this publication. Additionally, the editor acknowledges the support and collaboration provided by

Apple Academic Press, whose efforts were instrumental in the successful completion of this project.

—Prakash Kumar Sarangi, PhD
College of Agriculture,
Central Agricultural University,
Imphal, Manipur, India

CHAPTER 1

Bioprospective Fungi: Their Role and Importance in Sustainable Agriculture

KOTA CHAKRAPANI,[1] BIRESWAR SINHA,[2,*] BIJEETA THANGJAM,[1] W. TAMPAKLEIMA CHANU,[1] TUSI CHAKMA,[1] and PRAKASH KUMAR SARANGI[1]

[1]*College of Agriculture, Central Agricultural University, Imphal, Manipur, India*

[2]*Department of Plant Pathology, School of Agricultural Sciences, Nagaland University, Medziphema, Nagaland, India*

*Corresponding authors

ABSTRACT

The contemporary surge in population places significant stress on agriculture to fulfill daily sustenance requirements. This heightened demand exerts notable pressure, leading to the extensive application of chemical agents such as fertilizers and pesticides. Unfortunately, this widespread chemical use serves as a primary contributor to soil health degradation and environmental harm. Urgent attention is warranted to introduce eco-friendly methodologies as complementary measures for addressing prevailing agricultural challenges and initiating restoration processes. One promising avenue involves the incorporation of beneficial fungi into agricultural practices, offering sustainable management solutions. Various fungi possess the capacity to enhance plant health and foster growth. Additionally, they exhibit efficacy in disease suppression, mitigating substantial crop losses caused by various harmful pathogens. The multifaceted attributes of beneficial fungi, encompassing their roles as biofertilizers, biopesticides, and bioherbicides, collectively empower plants to withstand

Biotechnology for Sustainable Agriculture: Innovative Approaches and Strategies.
Prakash Kumar Sarangi (Ed)

DOI: 10.1201/9781779642998-1

a spectrum of biotic and abiotic stresses. This chapter delves into the significance of these fungi, elucidating their interactions within the soil and their role in restoring plant health. The insights provided contribute to the holistic enhancement of the agricultural sector.

1.1 INTRODUCTION

The global human population is poised to reach 9.7 billion, marking a 24% increase by 2050 (Desa, 2019). This substantial demographic surge places significant stress on the agricultural sector, which must augment food production by 70% to meet the escalating demands. Consequently, the agriculture sector resorts to the use of various hazardous chemicals to enhance production and satisfy the burgeoning population. The consumption of nitrogen (N) and phosphorus (P) fertilizers has witnessed a nine-fold and four-fold increase, respectively, contributing to cost-effective agricultural development (Schultz et al., 1995). While these chemicals yield positive impacts on production, they concurrently pose detrimental effects on soil health and the environment, introducing uncertainties. Furthermore, the production (in the Haber-Bosch process) and transportation (via fossil fuel combustion) of fertilizers lead to airborne carbon dioxide and nitrogen pollution, eventually deposited into terrestrial ecosystems. The prevalence of pre- and post-harvest diseases and pests compounds the challenges, necessitating increased chemical usage for management.

Nitrogen (N) and phosphorus (P) stand out as the most limiting nutrients for optimal plant growth. Nitrogen is intricately bound to soil organic matter. Post-fertilization, plants encounter competition with soil microbes for the acquisition of readily available soluble N. The challenges associated with phosphorus (P) differ, with phosphorus fertilizers proving ineffective in acidic soils despite supplementation in significant quantities. This ineffectiveness results from P fertilizers precipitating with iron, aluminum, and calcium phosphate in alkaline soils (Hinsinge, 2001). Consequently, overcoming P limitation poses a formidable challenge through the application of P-containing fertilizers.

The recent surge has been attributed to intensive agricultural practices. However, this increase comes at a substantial environmental cost. In contrast, developing countries face distinct challenges characterized by insufficient and inadequate fertilizers and agricultural practices. While the benefits of chemical use in agriculture are evident, the escalating drawbacks necessitate the exploration of novel approaches and methodologies to mitigate the adverse impacts of extensive chemical usage. This imperative has spurred researchers to devise innovative strategies. Clearly, there is an urgent global need for sustainable agricultural practices. In developed regions, a critical reduction in energy and environmental costs is imperative. In developing nations, the focus should be on implementing efficient and sustainable practices to enable cost-effective production of sufficient nutrition for burgeoning populations. Addressing ecological challenges arising from the depletion of plant nutrients and enhancing crop yields in the absence of resources for expensive fertilizers requires the adoption of sustainable solutions. Microscopic organisms that enhance nutrient utilization or increase nutrient availability offer promising avenues for present and future agricultural practices. Consequently, an enhanced understanding of the processes and factors governing the bioavailability of soil nutrients to plants, including insights into root-soil interactions and microorganisms in the rhizosphere (Martinez and Johnson, 2010), is crucial.

As highlighted by Samuil (2007), organic farming plays a pivotal role in promoting sustainable production systems characterized by diversified and balanced crops, aiming to prevent pollution and mitigate environmental damages. This underscores the importance of adopting environmentally conscious practices to ensure the long-term viability of agricultural systems. The inhabitants of the soil and rhizosphere, specifically fungi, serve as a valuable resource for effective nutrient management and the control of pests and diseases. These fungi play a crucial role in promoting plant growth by serving as a source of nutrition in an environmentally friendly manner. Certain fungi can be employed as an alternative strategy, enhancing both growth and defense mechanisms to combat a variety of disease-causing pathogens. Utilizing this plant growth-promoting bio-agents has the potential to minimize the need for chemical applications, offering protection against diverse pests and diseases.

Various fungi have been documented to enhance plant growth and fortify innate immunity, along with influencing essential secondary metabolites in plants (Hossain et al., 2017; Hyakumachi, 1994, 2004; Murali et al., 2012; Naziya et al., 2020). The beneficial effects facilitated by these fungi are mediated through mechanisms such as root colonization, growth hormone production, mineral solubilization, antagonism, mycoparasitism, and saprophytic resistance. These fungi foster nutritional competition and induce systemic resistance in plants, contributing to their overall health and resilience against various environmental stresses.

The advantageous effects facilitated by Plant Growth-Promoting Fungi (PGPF) stem from diverse mechanisms, including root colonization and growth hormone production. Additionally, PGPF induces systemic resistance (ISR) in plants (Meera et al., 1994; Shivanna et al., 2005; Whipps, 2001). Beyond their role in promoting growth, these fungi play a preventive role against plant infections, enhance nutrient availability in the soil, and mitigate the impact of toxic gases like ethylene. PGPF achieves this by producing 1-aminocyclopropane-1-carboxylate (ACC) deaminase and phytohormones (Naziya et al., 2020; Shoresh et al., 2005). This comprehensive overview underscores the significant role of PGPF in both promoting plant growth and fortifying plant resistance mechanisms. The plant growth and Endophyte Interactions.

PGPF play a pivotal role in promoting and modulating signaling hormones (Nawrocka et al., 2018; Tucci et al., 2011). Notably, PGPF induce the synthesis of elevated levels of secondary compounds such as lignin and callose. Concurrently, the fungi prompt the production of antioxidant enzymes, providing protection to the plant against various abiotic and anthropogenic stresses. These proactive measures are initiated prior to the regulation of defense signaling pathways.

1.2 BENEFICIAL ASPECTS OF PGPF

1.2.1 PRODUCTION OF PHYTOHORMONES

Phytohormones are pivotal in governing both the growth and defense mechanisms in plants. Among these hormones, Indole 3-acetic acid (IAA) stands out as one of the widely distributed natural auxins, predominantly enhancing root growth and morphology in plants (Hyakumachi and Kubota, 2004; Yadav et al., 2011). Utilizing sterile PGPF, specifically *Penicillium janczewskii*, has been noted to induce the production of IAA. This treatment demonstrated the ability to confer resistance against stem rot induced by *R. solani* by modifying the root growth of melon plants. While the involvement of auxin precursors in these phenomena remains undetermined, the enhanced root development aligns with the effects observed in fungal-mediated auxin production (Yadav et al., 2011).

Various soil-isolated species have been reported to produce and stimulate IAA in host plants, contributing to overall growth and yield enhancement (Abri et al., 2015; Kumar et al., 2017; Ozimek et al., 2018). Beyond IAA, another noteworthy phytohormone is gibberellic acid (GA), recognized as a diterpenoid acid. GA plays a crucial role in regulating seed germination, as well as the development of roots and shoots in plants. The multifaceted influence of these phytohormones underscores their significance in shaping various aspects of plant physiology and responses to environmental stimuli.

1.2.2 PLANT GROWTH PROMOTION

Distinct species of PGPF, including *Trichoderma, Talaromyces, Rhizoctonia, Aspergillus, Penicillium, Fusarium*, and others, have demonstrated positive effects on enhancing the growth of diverse crop plants (Dewan and Sivasithamparam, 1989; Meera et al., 1994; Murali et al., 2013; Shivanna et al., 2005). In a study by Shivanna et al. (2005), it was observed that specific *Penicillium* species (*P. janthinellum, P. citreonigrum*, and *P. citrinum*) residing in the rhizosphere of native *Zinnia* and tomato plants had a contrasting impact by inhibiting growth.

1.2.3 UPTAKE OF WATER

PGPF exhibit the capability to enhance the water economy of plants. The symbiotic mechanism employed by PGPF can either amplify the hydraulic conductivity of host plant roots, thereby improving water absorption, or modify the crop's physiology to reduce its response to water stress (Safir and Nelson, 1985). In instances of severe dry spells, plants associated with PGPF demonstrate superior endurance compared to those without such associations. Research suggests that the mycelial complex formed by these fungi may extend beneath and broaden the soil profile, exploring water and essential minerals. The fungal-plant association might also adjust the selectivity of the plasma membrane for water, enhancing phosphorus (P) nourishment and contributing to improved drought resistance (Osonubi et al., 1991; Sylvia and Williams, 1992).

Under water stress conditions, these fungi exert their influence by enhancing the transportational rate and promoting stomatal conductance through alterations in hormonal balance (Huang et al., 1985). Changes in leaf flexibility resulting from the association between fungi and plants improve water and turgor pressure in leaves, enhance root growth and extension, thereby influencing water relations and consequently, the water stress resistance of crops. The potential reasons behind the improved moisture and nutrient absorption in mycorrhiza-crop associations may be attributed to an enhanced allocation of the absorbing hyphal system, a more constructive ideotype of hyphae compared to roots, a superior absorbing area with a rapid expansion rate, improved functional longevity, chemical modifications in the soil rhizosphere influencing microorganisms inhabiting the sphere, altered uptake kinetics, superior hydraulic conductivities, reduced transportation rates per unit leaf area, and the withdrawal of moisture from the soil towards less Ψw and a more rapid recovery from moisture stress.

1.2.4 IMPROVEMENT OF SOIL TEXTURE AND STRUCTURE

Alterations in the ecological conditions exert a profound influence on the physical and biochemical dynamics of the soil. In the midst of this ecological disturbance, PGPF play a pivotal role by binding soil particles, thereby enhancing soil aggregation and contributing to soil conservation (Dodd, 2000). These fungi exhibit the capability to improve soil quality through the production of glomalin, which accumulates in the soil. Subsequently, the fungal hyphae contribute to the formation of microaggregates and, ultimately, macroaggregates, serving as the structural framework for soil aggregation and stabilization. Additionally, this process supports the proliferation of soil microbes.

1.3 RESISTANCE AGAINST STRESSORS

1.3.1 ANTAGONISM

This mechanism involves soil-resident fungi that actively inhibit the growth of invading pathogens, simultaneously promoting plant growth. The antagonistic attributes of PGPF stem from activities such as microbial predation, competition for nutrients, and the production of antibiotics (Mohiddin et al., 2017). Additionally, the antagonistic property may arise from the synthesis of lytic enzymes like protease, chitinase, and 1,3-glucanase (Benhamou et al., 1997). Numerous studies have identified various PGPF, including *T. harzianum*, *Phoma* sp., *F. equiseti*, and *P. simplicissimum*, as exhibiting antagonism against pathogens such as *R. solani*, *P. irregulare*, *S. rolfsii*, *F. oxysporum*, *P. syringae*, and *C. orbiculare*. Fungal predation, involving the activation of the chitinase gene, indirectly inhibits pathogen growth (Mohiddin et al., 2017).

Certain PGPF, like *Gliocladium virens*, produce antibiotics, such as *Gliovirin*, which restrict the growth of pathogens like *Pythium ultimum* (Gajera and Vakharia, 2012). While antagonism is often associated with the induction of resistance, reports suggest that it may not be the sole criterion. Various rhizospheric fungi, despite lacking antagonistic properties, have been found to induce resistance in plants against various pathogenic infections, indicating that factors beyond antagonism contribute to the resistance against pathogen attacks (Hyakumachi et al., 2004).

1.3.2 INDUCTION OF RESISTANCE

Induced resistance refers to the phenomenon of fortifying the plant's inherent immune system, activated by an inducer or elicitor effective against biotic stresses imposed by pathogens such as bacteria, viruses, and fungi (Choudhary et al., 2007; Hammerschmidt and Kuc, 1995). There are two primary forms of induced resistance: Induced Systemic Resistance (ISR) and Systemic Acquired Resistance (SAR), categorized based on the nature of the inducer and the associated signaling pathways (Sanchez-Montesinos et al., 2020). ISR employs an optimistic approach to reduce deleterious pathogens to zero levels. For instance, priming plant roots with PGPFs can systematically induce resistance in leaf and shoot areas, making it a safe and cost-effective method for enhancing crop plant growth and productivity (Howell et al., 1983; Toth et al., 2020).

Production of pathogenesis-related proteins (PRP) plays a pivotal role in bolstering the plant's defense system against invading pathogens (Hunt and Ryals, 1996). In tobacco plants, SAR activation significantly reduces the occurrence of disease symptoms induced by various pathogenic microbes, including *Phytophthora parasitica*, *Cercospora nicotianae*, *Peronospora tabacina*, *Tobacco mosaic virus* pv. *tabaci* (TMV), *P. Syringae*, *Tobacco necrosis virus* (TNV), and *Erwinia carotovora* (Neuenschwander et al., 1995).

1.3.3 *MORPHOLOGICAL AND HISTOCHEMICAL DEFENSE*

The primary barrier to gain access to the host plant for an invading pathogen is the cell wall, which plays a pivotal role in defense. The invading pathogen must breach the host plant's cell wall before entering. Treatment with PGPF fortifies the cell wall by increasing the deposition of wall materials, forming a robust defensive barrier. These wall materials primarily consist of phenol, lignin, and callose (Hossain et al., 2017; Hyakumachi and Kubota, 2004).

To withstand deleterious pathogens, plants develop a resistance mechanism involving hypersensitive reactions (HR) and the biosynthesis of antibiotics, including phytoalexins, to impart resistance. HR results in localized necrosis, that is, cell death of plant cells occurring at the site of infection, limiting the invading pathogen and preventing further spread (Darvill and Albersheim, 1984). The initial event in HR is the rapid production of reactive oxygen species (ROS) compounds, leading to the generation of ROS like hydroxyl radicals, superoxide, and hydrogen peroxide (H_2O_2) (Sequeira, 1983). The deposition of H_2O_2 in cell membranes due to ROS at the infection site inhibits the growth and development of the invading pathogen (Heath, 1997). ROS production is toxic and has lethal effects on both microorganisms and the plant's own cells. Various antioxidant enzymes, whose activity is elevated upon PGPF treatment under biotic and abiotic stress, effectively induce increased ROS, impacting the plant's own cells and causing Programmed Cell Death. Callose deposition occurs during resistance interactions upon pathogen infection, and it can also take place during pre-treatment with certain chemicals or biotic inducers, eliciting the innate protective resistance mechanism in plants (Koge et al., 1994; Lamb and Dixon, 1997).

Lignin, a secondary metabolite produced in plant cells via the phenylalanine/tyrosine metabolic pathway, acts as a potential barrier against deleterious pathogens. It triggers plant defense upon pathogen entry by depositing lignin across the entire cell wall, on a set of cells, or specifically at the site of pathogen infection (Siddaiah et al., 2017).

1.3.4 *BIOCHEMICAL DEFENSE*

The innate immunity of plants involves biochemical mechanisms that come into play when the plant is invaded by a pathogen. In addition to morphological and histological changes, biochemical alterations occur at the point of interaction between the pathogen and the host. This interaction induces changes in cell metabolism and enzyme activities, including phenylalanine ammonia-lyase (PAL), peroxidase (POX), lipoxygenase (LOX), superoxide dismutase (SOD), β-1,3 glucans, and polyphenol oxidase (PPO) (Muslim et al., 2017).

The seed treatment with specific types of PGPF, such as *Rhizoctonia* sp., *Fusarium* sp., *Aspergillus* sp., *Phoma* spp., *Talaromyces* spp., *Trichoderma* sp., *Pythium* sp., *Penicillium* sp., and non-sporulating fungi, has been shown to enhance the occurrence rates of peroxidase (POX) in cucumber, pearl millet, and chili.

1.3.5 PGPF IN ABIOTIC STRESS IMPROVEMENT

Crop plants often face a diverse array of abiotic stresses, including elevated temperatures, drought, salinity, floods, and heavy metal accumulation, significantly impacting their overall production. A substantial portion of cultivated land experiences at least one of the aforementioned stresses, potentially resulting in a significant 70% reduction in yield (Mantri, 2007; Sanchez-Montesinos et al., 2019). Cereal crops, in particular, are under considerable threat from climate change, posing a substantial risk to global food security. The prevalence of saline content in cultivated lands has reached up to 37% between 1990 and 2013 (Tigchelaar et al., 2018).

The growth promotion mediated by PGPF in plants under stressful conditions is attributed to alterations in root architecture, the solubilization of minerals from decomposed organic matter, and the production of secondary metabolites. Naturally occurring PGPF in soil systems possess the inherent ability to fortify the plant's immune system and enhance overall plant growth when subjected to challenging environmental conditions.

1.3.6 PGPF AS A SOURCE OF ALTERNATIVE

Plant-microbe interactions extend beyond disease outcomes, encompassing various defense mechanisms employed by plants at both local and systemic levels. Numerous mutually beneficial relationships between plants and microbes play a crucial role in agricultural productivity and overall plant health, attracting extensive research attention. In symbiotic associations, microbes aid in nutrient absorption or contribute biochemical and molecular activities lacking in the plant, while the plant reciprocates by providing photosynthate, conferring a competitive advantage to the microbial symbiont in the rhizosphere. Symbiotic associations can also alter the rhizosphere's microflora balance, potentially safeguarding plants from disease-causing microbes (Naziya et al., 2020).

While current research predominantly focuses on combatting plant diseases through chemical insecticides, pesticides, and fungicides, these substances pose threats to beneficial soil microflora and are not considered safe for human consumption. Additionally, the application of chemical fertilizers, particularly nitrogen (N), phosphorus (P), and potassium (K), for enhancing crop growth leads to soil pollution (Pang et al., 2020). Consequently, research communities have proposed eco-friendly strategies over the last decade to reduce reliance on chemical-based fertilizers in crop improvement and management studies. Biocontrol agents such as endophytes, Arbuscular mycorrhizae (AM) fungi, plant extracts, and Plant Growth-Promoting Rhizobacteria (PGPR) have gained attention as substitutes for controlling plant diseases caused by harmful microbes (Gowtham et al., 2020; Savci, 2012).

Among these, PGPF emerges as a relatively underexplored but promising eco-friendly source for combatting bacterial and fungal diseases in plants. PGPF plays a crucial role in enhancing plant growth, fruit yield, nutrient composition, and bolstering plants' immunity by reinforcing their defense machinery to regulate pathogen infections. To date, the exploration of PGPFs holds promise as a viable alternative to contemporary practices and warrants further investigation for sustainable agriculture.

1.4 CONCLUSION AND FUTURE PROSPECTS

Bio prospective fungi, with their diverse roles and significant contributions, play a pivotal role in advancing the cause of sustainable agriculture. The exploration of fungi for their potential in enhancing agricultural practices is gaining prominence due to the urgent need for environmentally friendly alternatives. In this conclusion, we delve into the multifaceted contributions of bio prospective fungi, emphasizing their importance in sustainable agriculture.

One of the key aspects of bio prospective fungi is their ability to establish symbiotic relationships with plants. These mutually beneficial associations, often formed in the rhizosphere, contribute to nutrient uptake, root development, and overall plant health. Fungi have been extensively studied for their positive effects on crop productivity. The mycorrhizal symbiosis enhances nutrient absorption, particularly phosphorus, facilitating the plant's adaptation to nutrient-limiting conditions. PGPR, on the other hand, contribute to plant growth promotion through various mechanisms, including the production of phytohormones and the solubilization of minerals.

Moreover, bio prospective fungi showcase their prowess in disease management. In contrast to conventional methods relying on chemical pesticides, which pose environmental and health risks, fungi offer a sustainable alternative. Antagonistic relationships between fungi and plant pathogens, as well as the induction of systemic resistance in plants, form the basis of biocontrol strategies. Fungi such as *Trichoderma*, *Penicillium*, and *Fusarium* have demonstrated their efficacy in suppressing various plant diseases, offering a more sustainable approach to pest and pathogen management. In the context of the burgeoning global population, the demand for increased food production is escalating. Bio prospective fungi emerge as valuable allies in addressing this challenge. Their ability to enhance nutrient availability, stimulate plant growth, and protect against diseases contributes to improved crop yields. The ecological impact of agricultural practices is a critical consideration in the pursuit of sustainability. Bio prospective fungi contribute to soil health by promoting aggregation, enhancing water retention, and participating in nutrient cycling. The secretion of glomalin and the formation of micro and macroaggregates by fungal hyphae contribute to soil structure and stability. Additionally, the role of fungi in the decomposition of organic matter contributes to the overall fertility of the soil, reducing dependence on external inputs.

In the face of climate change, characterized by unpredictable weather patterns, extreme temperatures, and altered precipitation, resilient agricultural practices are imperative. The intricate mechanisms involved in stress response, including the synthesis of osmoprotectants and the modulation of antioxidant enzymes, showcase the adaptability of plants under the influence of beneficial fungi. A significant advantage of bio prospective fungi is their eco-friendly nature. Unlike chemical inputs that often lead to soil and water pollution, fungi promote sustainable agricultural practices. The reduced reliance on synthetic fertilizers and pesticides mitigates the environmental impact associated with conventional agriculture. This aligns with the global movement towards more sustainable and ecologically conscious farming methods. The potential of bio prospective fungi extends beyond their direct interactions with plants. They contribute to the overall biodiversity of soil ecosystems by influencing the composition of microbial communities. This biodiversity, in turn, has cascading effects on nutrient cycling, soil structure, and the overall resilience of ecosystems. Fungi, acting as ecosystem engineers, shape the dynamics of the soil environment, creating conditions conducive to plant growth and vitality.

In conclusion, bio prospective fungi represent a cornerstone in the edifice of sustainable agriculture. Their multifaceted roles encompass nutrient cycling, disease management, stress tolerance, and soil health promotion. As we navigate the complexities of modern agriculture and grapple with the challenges of a changing climate, harnessing the potential of these fungi becomes imperative. By integrating bio prospective fungi into agricultural practices, we can foster a resilient, environmentally friendly, and sustainable approach to food production. The ongoing research in this field holds promise for unlocking further insights into the intricate relationships between fungi, plants, and the environment, paving the way for a more sustainable and harmonious coexistence between agriculture and nature.

KEYWORDS

- **agricultural practices**
- **bioprospective fungi**
- **nutrient cycling**
- **osmoprotectants**
- **sustainable agriculture**
- **water retention**

REFERENCES

Abri, T. K., Sengin, E. L., & Sjahrir, R. (2015). Production of indole acetic acid (IAA) hormone from fungal isolates collected from rhizosphere of aromatic rice in Tana Toraja. *International Journal of Current Research in Biosciences and Plant Biology, 2*, 198–201.

Albrechtová, J., Látr, A., Nedorost, L., Pokluda, R., Pošta, K., & Vosátka, M. (2012). Dual inoculation with mycorrhizal and saprotrophic fungi applicable in sustainable cultivation improves the yield and nutritive value of onion. *Scientific World Journal, 2012*, 1–8.

Al-Waily, D. S., & Hassan, S. M. (2019). Effect of two bioformulation *Trichoderma harzianum* and *Pseudomonas fluorescens* with manure in controlling *Fusarium* wilt disease in pumpkin. *Journal of University of Babylon for Pure and Applied Sciences, 27*, 446–456.

Arnold, A. E., & Engelbrecht, B. M. J. (2007). Fungal endophytes nearly double minimum leaf conductance in seedlings of a neotropical tree species. *Journal of Tropical Ecology, 23*, 369–372.

Benhamou, N., & Chet, I. (2017). Cellular and molecular mechanisms involved in the interaction between *Trichoderma harzianum* and *Pythium ultimum*. *Applied and Environmental Microbiology, 63*, 2095–2099.

Chalot, M., & Brun, A. (1998). Physiology of organic nitrogen acquisition by ectomycorrhizal fungi and ectomycorrhizas. *FEMS Microbiology Reviews, 22*, 21–44.

Chandanie, W. A., Kubota, M., & Hyakumachi, M. (2009). Interactions between arbuscular mycorrhizal fungus *Glomus mosseae* and plant growth promoting fungi and their significance for enhancing plant growth and suppressing damping-off of cucumber (*Cucumis sativus* L.). *Applied Soil Ecology, 41*, 336–341.

Chang, Y. C., Baker, R., Kleifeld, O., & Chet, I. (1986). Increased growth of plants in the presence of the biological control agent *Trichoderma harzianum*. *Plant Disease, 70*, 145–148.

Chaverri, P., & Gazis, R. O. (2010). *Perisporiopsis lateritia*, a new species on decaying leaves of *Hevea* spp. from the Amazon basin in Peru. *Mycotaxon, 113*, 163–169.

Choudhary, D. K., Prakash, A., & Johri, B. N. (2007). Induced systemic resistance (ISR) in plants: Mechanism of action. *Indian Journal of Microbiology, 47*, 289–297.

Cohen, R., Persky, L., & Hadar, Y. (2002). Biotechnological applications and potential of wood-degrading mushrooms of the genus *Pleurotus*. *Applied Microbiology and Biotechnology, 58*, 582–594.

Contreras-Cornejo, H. A., Macias-Rodriguez, L., Cortes-Penagos, C., & Lopez-Bucio, J. (2009). *Trichoderma virens*, a plant beneficial fungus, enhances biomass production and promotes lateral root growth through an auxin-dependent mechanism in *Arabidopsis*. *Plant Physiology* (American Society of Plant Biologists), *149*, 1579–1592.

Darvill, A. G., & Albersheim, P. (1984). Phytoalexins and their elicitors: A defense against microbial infection in plants. *Annual Review of Plant Physiology, 35*, 243–275.

Desa, U. N. (2019). *World Population Prospects 2019: Highlights*. United Nations Department for Economic and Social Affairs: New York, NY, USA. https://www.un.org/development/desa/publications/world-population-prospects-2019-highlights.html (accessed on 2nd January 2026).

Dewan, M., & Sivasithamparam, K. (1989). Growth promotion of rotation crop species by sterile fungus from wheat and effect of soil temperature and water potential on its suppression of take-all. *Mycological Research, 93*, 156–160.

Dodd, J. C. (2000). The role of arbuscular mycorrhizal fungi in natural ecosystems. *Outlook on Agriculture, 29*(1), 55–62.

Gajera, H. P., & Vakharia, D. N. (2012). Production of lytic enzymes by *Trichoderma* isolates during *in vitro* antagonism with *Aspergillus niger*, the causal agent of collar rot of peanut. *Brazilian Journal of Microbiology, 43*, 43–52.

Gowtham, H. G., Singh, B., Murali, M., Shilpa, N., Prasad, M., Aiyaz, M., Amruthesh, K. N., & Niranjana, S. R. (2020). Induction of drought tolerance in tomato upon the application of ACC deaminase producing plant growth promoting rhizobacterium *Bacillus subtilis* Rhizo SF 48. *Microbiological Research, 234*, 126422.

Ha, T. N. (2010). Using *Trichoderma* species for biological control of plant pathogens in Vietnam. *Journal of the International Society for Southeast Asian Agricultural Sciences, 16*, 17–21.

Hamayun, M., Khan, S. A., Khan, M. A., Khan, A. L., Kang, S. M., Kim, S. K., Joo, G. J., & Lee, I. J. (2009). Gibberellin production by pure cultures of a new strain of *Aspergillus fumigatus*. *World Journal of Microbiology and Biotechnology, 25*, 1785–1792.

Hammerschmidt, R., & Kuc, J. (1995). *Induced Resistance to Disease in Plants*. Kluwer: Dordrecht, The Netherlands, p. 182.

Harman, G., & Mastouri, F. (2010). The role of *Trichoderma* in crop management systems. *Phytopathology, 100*, 16.

Heath, M. C. (1997). Hypersensitive response-related death. *Plant Molecular Biology, 44*, 321–334.

Hinsinger, P. (2001). Bioavailability of trace elements as related to root-induced chemical changes in the rhizosphere. In Gobran, G. K., Wenzel, W. W., & Lombi, E. (Eds.), *Trace Elements in the Rhizosphere* (pp. 25–41). CRC Press LCC: Boca Raton, Florida, USA.

Hodge, A., Campbell, C. D., Fitter, A. H., et al. (2001). An arbuscular mycorrhizal fungus accelerates decomposition and acquires nitrogen directly from organic matter. *Nature, 413*, 297–299.

Hoorman, J. J. (2011). *The Role of Soil Fungus* (Report No. SAG-14-11). Columbus, Ohio, USA: Ohio State University.

Horinouchi, H., Katsuyama, N., Taguchi, Y., & Hyakumachi, M. (2008). Control of *Fusarium* crown and root rot of tomato in a soil system by combination of a plant growth-promoting fungus, *Fusarium equiseti*, and biodegradable pots. *Crop Protection, 27*, 859–864.

Hossain, M. M., Sultana, F., & Islam, S. (2017). Plant growth-promoting fungi (PGPF): Phytostimulation and induced systemic resistance. In *Plant-Microbe Interactions in Agro-Ecological Perspectives* (pp. 135–191). Springer: Singapore.

Hossain, M. M., Sultana, F., & Islam, S. (2020). Plant growth-promoting fungi (PGPF): Phytostimulation and induced systemic resistance. In *Plant-Microbe Interactions in Agro-Ecological Perspectives* (pp. 135–191). Springer: Singapore.

Howell, C. R., & Stipanovic, R. D. (1983). Gliovirin, a new antibiotic from *Gliocladium virens* and its role in the biological control of *Pythium ultimum*. *Canadian Journal of Microbiology, 29*, 321–324.

Huang, R. S., Smith, W. K., & Yost, R. E. (1985). Influence of vesicular-arbuscular mycorrhizae on growth, water relation, and leaf orientation in *Leucaena leucocephala* (Linn.) De Wit. *New Phytologist, 99*, 229–243.

Hunt, M., & Ryals, J. (1996). Systemic acquired resistance signal transduction. *Critical Reviews in Plant Sciences, 15*, 583–606.

Hyakumachi, M. (1994). Plant-growth-promoting fungi from turfgrass rhizosphere with potential for disease suppression. *Soil Microorganisms, 44*, 53–68.

Hyakumachi, M., & Kubota, M. (2004). Fungi as plant growth promoter and disease suppressor. *Fungal Biotechnology in Agricultural, Food and Environmental Applications, 21*, 101–110.

Kaur, R., Kaur, J., & Singh, R. S. (2011). Non-pathogenic *Fusarium* as a biological control agent. *Plant Pathology Journal, 9*, 79–91.

Khan, S. A., Hamayun, M., Yoon, H., Kim, H. Y., Suh, S. J., Hwang, S. K., Kim, J. M., Lee, I. J., Choo, Y. S., Yoon, U. H., et al. (2008). Plant growth promotion and *Penicillium citrinum*. *BMC Microbiology, 8*, 231.

Kogel, K. H., Beckhove, U., Dreschers, J., Munch, S., & Romme, Y. (1994). Acquired resistance in barley: The resistance mechanism induced by 2,6-dichloroisonicotinic acid is a phenocopy of a genetically based mechanism governing race-specific powdery mildew resistance. *Plant Physiology, 106*, 1269–1277.

Kumar, N. V., Rajam, K. S., & Rani, M. E. (2017). Plant growth promotion efficacy of indole acetic acid (IAA) produced by a mangrove-associated fungi–*Trichoderma viride* VKF3. *International Journal of Current Microbiology and Applied Sciences, 6*, 2692–2701.

Lamb, C., & Dixon, R. A. (1997). The oxidative burst in plant disease resistance. *Annual Review of Plant Physiology and Plant Molecular Biology, 48*, 251–275.

Lindsey, D. L., & Baker, R. (1967). Effect of certain fungi on dwarf tomatoes grown under gnotobiotic conditions. *Phytopathology, 57*, 1262–1263.

Mantri, N. L., Ford, R., Coram, T. E., & Pang, E. C. K. (2007). Transcriptional profiling of chickpea genes differentially regulated in response to high-salinity, cold and drought. *BMC Genomics, 8*, 303.

Martinez, T. N., & Johnson, N. C. (2010). Agricultural management influences propagule densities and functioning of arbuscular mycorrhizas in low and high input agroecosystems in arid environment. *Applied Soil Ecology, 46*(2), 300–306.

Meera, M. S., Shivanna, M. B., Kageyama, K., & Hyakumachi, M. (1994). Plant growth promoting fungi from zoysiagrass rhizosphere as potential inducers of systemic resistance in cucumbers. *Phytopathology, 84*, 1399–1406.

Mohiddin, F. A., Bashir, I., Padder, S. A., & Hamid, B. (2017). Evaluation of different substrates for mass multiplication of *Trichoderma* species. *Journal of Pharmacognosy and Phytochemistry, 6*, 563–569.

Murali, M., Amruthesh, K. N., Sudisha, J., Niranjana, S. R., & Shetty, H. S. (2012). Screening for plant growth promoting fungi and their ability for growth promotion and induction of resistance in pearl millet against downy mildew disease. *Journal of Phytology, 4*, 30–36.

Murali, M., Naziya, B., Ansari, M. A., Alomary, M. N., AlYahya, S., Almatroudi, A., Thriveni, M. C., Gowtham, H. G., Singh, S. B., Aiyaz, M., et al. (2021). Bioprospecting of rhizosphere-resident fungi: Their role and importance in sustainable agriculture. *Journal of Fungi, 7*, 314.

Murali, M., Sudisha, J., Amruthesh, K. N., & Shetty, H. S. (2013). Rhizosphere fungus *Penicillium chrysogenum* promotes growth and induces defence-related genes and downy mildew disease resistance in pearl millet. *Plant Biology, 15*, 111–118.

Muslim, A., Hyakumachi, M., Kageyama, K., & Suwandi, S. (2019). Induction of systemic resistance in cucumber by hypovirulent binucleate *Rhizoctonia* against anthracnose caused by *Colletotrichum orbiculare*. *Tropical Life Sciences Research, 30*, 109.

Nawrocka, J., Małolepsza, U., Szymczak, K., & Szczech, M. (2018). Involvement of metabolic components, volatile compounds, PR proteins, and mechanical strengthening in multilayer protection of cucumber plants against *Rhizoctonia solani* activated by *Trichoderma atroviride* TRS25. *Protoplasma, 255*, 359–373.

Naziya, B., Murali, M., & Amruthesh, K. N. (2020). Plant growth-promoting fungi (PGPF) instigate plant growth and induce disease resistance in *Capsicum annuum* L. upon infection with *Colletotrichum capsici* (Syd.) Butl. Bisby. *Biomolecules, 10*, 41.

Neuenschwander, U., Friedrich, L., Delaney, T., Vernooij, B., Kessmann, H., & Ryals, J. (1995). Activation of plant disease resistance. *Aspects of Applied Biology, 42*, 217–225.

Osonubi, O., Mulongoy, K., Awotoye, O. O., Atayese, M. O., & Okali, D. V. V. (1991). Effect of ectomycorrhizal and vesicular-arbuscular mycorrhizal fungi on drought tolerance of four leguminous woody seedlings. *Plant and Soil, 136*, 131–143.

Ozimek, E., Jaroszuk-Sciseł, J., Bohacz, J., Korniłłowicz-Kowalska, T., Tyskiewicz, R., Słomka, A., Nowak, A., & Hanaka, A. (2018). Synthesis of indole acetic acid, gibberellic acid and ACC-deaminase by *Mortierella* strains promote winter wheat seedlings growth under different conditions. *International Journal of Molecular Sciences, 19*, 3218.

Pang, Z., Zhao, Y., Xu, P., & Yu, D. (2020). Microbial diversity of upland rice roots and their influence on rice growth and drought tolerance. *Microorganisms, 8*, 1329.

Phillips, R. P., Meier, I. C., Bernhardt, E. S., Grandy, S., Wickings, K., & Finzi, A. C. (2012). Roots and fungi accelerate carbon and nitrogen cycling in forests exposed to elevated CO_2. *Ecology Letters, 15*, 1042–1049.

Safir, G. R., & Nelson, C. E. (1985). VA-mycorrhizas: Plant and fungal water relations. In Molina, R. (Ed.), *Proceedings of the 6th North American Conference on Mycorrhiza* (p. 471). Corvallis.

Samuil, C. (2007). *Tehnologii de Agricultură Ecologică*. U.S.A.M.V. Iaşi.

Sanchez-Montesinos, B., Dianez, F., Moreno-Gavira, A., Gea, F. J., & Santos, M. (2019). Plant growth promotion and biocontrol of *Pythium ultimum* by saline tolerant *Trichoderma* isolates under salinity stress. *International Journal of Environmental Research and Public Health, 16*, 2053.

Sanchez-Montesinos, B., Dianez, F., Moreno-Gavira, A., Gea, F. J., & Santos, M. (2020). Role of *Trichoderma aggressivum* f. *europaeum* as plant-growth promoter in horticulture. *Agronomy, 10*, 1004.

Savci, S. (2012). An agricultural pollutant: Chemical fertilizer. *International Journal of Environmental Science and Development, 3*, 73.

Schultz, R. C., Colletti, J. P., Isenhart, T. M., Simkins, W. W., Mize, C. W., & Thompson, M. L. (1995). Design and placement of a multi-species riparian buffer strip system. *Agroforestry Systems, 29*, 1–16.

Sequeira, L. (1983). Mechanisms of induced resistance in plants. *Annual Review of Microbiology, 37*, 51–79.

Shanmugaiah, V., Mathivanan, N., & Varghese, B. (2010). Purification, crystal structure and antimicrobial activity of phenazine-1-carboxamide produced by a growth-promoting biocontrol bacterium, *Pseudomonas aeruginosa* MML2212. *Journal of Applied Microbiology, 108*, 703–711.

Shivanna, M. B., Meera, M. S., Kubota, M., & Hyakumachi, M. (2005). Promotion of growth and yield in cucumber by zoysia grass rhizosphere fungi. *Microbes and Environments, 20*, 34–40.

Shoresh, M., Yedidia, I., & Chet, I. (2005). Involvement of jasmonic acid/ethylene signaling pathway in the systemic resistance induced in cucumber by *Trichoderma asperellum* T203. *Phytopathology*, *95*, 76–84.

Siddaiah, C. N., Satyanarayana, N. R., Mudili, V., Gupta, V. K., Gurunathan, S., Rangappa, S., Huntrike, S. S., & Srivastava, R. K. (2017). Elicitation of resistance and associated defense responses in *Trichoderma hamatum*-induced protection against pearl millet downy mildew pathogen. *Scientific Reports*, *7*, 43991.

Sylvia, D. M., & Williams, S. E. (1992). Mycorrhizae and environmental stresses. In Bethlenfalvay, G. J., & Linderman, R. G. (Eds.), *Mycorrhizae in Sustainable Agriculture* (ASA Special Publication No. 54, pp. 101–124). Madison, WI.

Tigchelaar, M., Battisti, D. S., Naylor, R. L., & Ray, D. K. (2018). Future warming increases probability of globally synchronized maize production shocks. *Proceedings of the National Academy of Sciences of the United States of America*, *115*, 6644–6649.

Toth, L., Varadi, G., Boros, E., Borics, A., Ficze, H., Nagy, I., Toth, G. K., Rakhely, G., Marx, F., & Galgoczy, L. (2020). Biofungicidal potential of *Neosartorya (Aspergillus) fischeri* antifungal protein NFAP and novel synthetic γ-core peptides. *Frontiers in Microbiology*, *11*, 820.

Tucci, M., Ruocco, M., De Masi, L., De Palma, M., & Lorito, M. (2011). The beneficial effect of *Trichoderma* spp. on tomato is modulated by plant genotype. *Molecular Plant Pathology*, *12*, 341–354.

Wakelin, S. A., Gupta, V. V. S. R., Harvey, P. R., & Ryder, M. H. (2007). The effect of *Penicillium* fungi on plant growth and phosphorus mobilization in neutral to alkaline soils from southern Australia. *Canadian Journal of Microbiology*, *53*, 106–115.

Wells, J. M., Boddy, L., & Donnelly, D. P. (1998). Wood decay and phosphorus translocation by the cord-forming basidiomycete *Phanerochaete velutina*: The significance of local nutrient supply. *The New Phytologist*, *138*, 607–617.

Whipps, J. M. (2001). Microbial interactions and biocontrol in the rhizosphere. *Journal of Experimental Botany*, *52*, 487–511.

Windham, M. T., Elad, Y., & Baker, R. (1986). A mechanism for increased plant growth induced by *Trichoderma* spp. *Phytopathology*, *76*, 518–521.

Yadav, J., Verma, J. P., & Tiwari, K. N. (2011). Plant growth promoting activities of fungi and their effect on chickpea plant growth. *Asian Journal of Biological Sciences*, *4*, 291–299.

Yadav, R. L., Shukla, S. K., Suman, A., & Singh, P. N. (2009). *Trichoderma* inoculation and trash management effects on soil microbial biomass, soil respiration, nutrient uptake and yield of ratoon sugarcane under subtropical conditions. *Biology and Fertility of Soils*, *45*, 461–468.

Yaseen, T., Burni, T., & Hussain, F. (2011). Effect of arbuscular mycorrhizal inoculation on nutrient uptake, growth and productivity of cowpea (*Vigna unguiculata*) varieties. *African Journal of Biotechnology*, *10*, 8593–8598.

Zhang, F., Huo, Y., Cobb, A. B., Luo, G., Zhou, J., Yang, G., Wilson, G. W., & Zhang, Y. (2018). *Trichoderma* biofertilizer links to altered soil chemistry, altered microbial communities, and improved grassland biomass. *Frontiers in Microbiology*, *9*, 848.

CHAPTER 2

Plant Growth-Promoting Rhizobacteria: Innovations in Agricultural Sustainability

PRITI PAL,[1] AKHILESH KUMAR SINGH,[2] OM PRAKASH,[2] UTTAM KUMAR SAHOO,[3,*] ANAND PRAKASH,[2] BRIJESH PANDEY,[2] RAHUL GUPTA,[1] and PRAKASH KUMAR SARANGI[4]

[1]*Amity Institute of Biotechnology, Amity University Uttar Pradesh, Lucknow Campus, Lucknow, Uttar Pradesh, India*

[2]*Department of Biotechnology, School of Life Sciences, Mahatma Gandhi Central University, Motihari, Bihar, India*

[3]*Department of Forestry, Mizoram University, Aizawl, Mizoram, India*

[4]*College of Agriculture, Central Agricultural University, Imphal, Manipur, India*

*Corresponding authors

ABSTRACT

In the face of burgeoning global agricultural challenges, sustainable practices are imperative to ensure food security and environmental stewardship. Plant growth-promoting rhizobacteria (PGPR) have emerged as key contributors to agricultural sustainability, offering multifaceted benefits to plants and the ecosystem. This abstract provides a succinct overview of the pivotal role that PGPR plays in enhancing plant growth, nutrient availability, and stress tolerance. PGPR-mediated plant growth promotion is intricately linked to their ability to produce phytohormones,

Biotechnology for Sustainable Agriculture: Innovative Approaches and Strategies.
Prakash Kumar Sarangi (Ed)

DOI: 10.1201/9781779642998-2

facilitate nutrient solubilization, and induce systemic resistance. An eco-friendly alternative to synthetic agrochemicals. PGPR applications alleviate the environmental footprint of traditional farming methods. By diminishing dependence on synthetic fertilizers and pesticides, PGPR harmonizes with the worldwide transition towards sustainable and eco-friendly agriculture. The positive influence of PGPR on soil structure and microbial communities further underscores its role in fostering resilient and sustainable agroecosystems. This abstract emphasizes the need for continued research to unlock the full potential of PGPR in sustainable agriculture. By harnessing the biological prowess of these beneficial rhizobacteria, farmers can optimize resource utilization, minimize environmental degradation, and enhance overall agricultural productivity.

2.1 INTRODUCTION

In the midst of the 21st century, global agriculture finds itself at a crossroads, facing the formidable challenge of feeding a burgeoning population amidst escalating environmental concerns. Conventional agricultural practices, characterized by intensive use of synthetic fertilizers and pesticides, extensive tillage, and mono-cropping, have significantly contributed to soil degradation, loss of biodiversity, and environmental pollution. As the ecological impact of agriculture becomes more evident, there is a rising acknowledgment of the pressing necessity to pivot towards farming methods that are both sustainable and environmentally sound. In this evolving landscape, the rhizosphere, the dynamic interface between plant roots and the soil, has emerged as a focal point for exploring innovative and sustainable agricultural solutions. Within this intricate microcosm, a group of microorganisms known as Plant Growth-Promoting Rhizobacteria (PGPR) has taken center stage. These bacteria, encompassing genera such as *Bacillus, Pseudomonas,* and *Rhizobium*, form symbiotic relationships with plant roots, exerting profound influences on plant health, growth, and resilience to environmental stressors.

At the forefront of sustainable agriculture, PGPR's pivotal role shines through its capacity to augment plant growth via the synthesis of phytohormones. Phytohormones, such as auxins, cytokinin's, and gibberellins, play pivotal roles in regulating plant development and growth.

PGPR contribute to the plant's hormonal milieu, promoting root and shoot development, increased branching, and overall plant vigor. This natural and targeted approach to promoting plant growth stands in stark contrast to the indiscriminate use of synthetic growth regulators and fertilizers in conventional agriculture. Furthermore, PGPR play indispensable roles in nutrient cycling and stewardship. Engaging in activities like nitrogen fixation and phosphorus solubilization, these microorganisms elevate the accessibility of vital nutrients for plant uptake. Notably, nitrogen-fixing bacteria such as those within the *Rhizobium* genus establish symbiotic partnerships with leguminous flora, transforming atmospheric nitrogen into a usable form for plants. This reduces the need for synthetic nitrogen fertilizers, mitigating the environmental impact associated with their production and application.

Phosphorus, an essential nutrient for plant development, frequently exists in insoluble states within the soil. However, PGPR, by excreting phosphatase enzymes and organic acids, mobilize phosphorus, rendering it more readily available for plant uptake. This phosphorus solubilization capability not only enhances nutrient uptake but also reduces the reliance on phosphorus-containing fertilizers, addressing concerns related to eutrophication and phosphate rock depletion. In addition to nutrient management, PGPR are potent modulators of plant defense mechanisms. The rhizosphere, despite being a zone of mutualistic interactions, is not immune to potential threats from pathogenic microbes. PGPR, however, deploy an array of strategies to confer systemic resistance to plants against pathogenic invaders.

This entails triggering systemic acquired resistance (SAR) and induced systemic resistance (ISR), whereby the plant's inherent defense mechanisms are primed to mount stronger responses against future pathogenic assaults. The ability of PGPR to enhance plant resilience is particularly crucial in the context of climate change and its associated abiotic stresses. Drought, salinity, and temperature extremes are becoming increasingly prevalent, posing significant challenges to global agriculture. PGPR, through the production of stress-responsive proteins, osmoprotectants, and enzymes, assist plants in acclimating to and surviving under adverse environmental conditions. This stress mitigation capacity not only ensures the stability of crop yields but also reduces the need for water-intensive irrigation practices.

As the global agricultural community seeks sustainable alternatives, PGPR offer a compelling solution by promoting environmental stewardship and resilience. By reducing the reliance on synthetic agrochemicals, PGPR play a role in maintaining soil vitality, upholding water purity, and ensuring the overall integrity of ecosystems. Moreover, the positive impact of PGPR extends beyond individual plants to entire agroecosystems, fostering biodiversity and ecological balance. The potential of PGPR is not limited to theoretical promise; practical applications in diverse cropping systems underscore their efficacy. Numerous studies have demonstrated the benefits of PGPR inoculation in various crops, ranging from staple grains like rice and wheat to cash crops like cotton and vegetables. Inoculation with PGPR has been shown to enhance crop yields, improve nutrient content, and confer resistance against a spectrum of pathogens. Though the benefits of PGPR in sustainable farming are clear, effectively integrating these strategies demands a deep comprehension of the intricate dynamics within the rhizosphere. Factors such as soil type, plant species, and environmental conditions influence the effectiveness of PGPR-based interventions. Moreover, considerations related to the selection of optimal PGPR strains, their compatibility with specific crops, and the development of suitable formulations for application in diverse agricultural contexts are critical aspects that demand attention.

In summary, the contribution of PGPR to sustainable agriculture is diverse, covering aspects such as promoting plant growth, managing nutrients, enhancing stress tolerance, and controlling diseases. These bacteria, acting as natural partners to plants, offer an enticing departure from conventional farming methods that frequently lead to environmental harm. Embracing the capabilities of PGPR signifies a shift towards a more comprehensive and environmentally aware farming approach. Amidst the global struggle to ensure food security amidst climate change, PGPR emerge as promising companions in the pursuit of sustainable and adaptable agriculture.

2.2 SOIL FERTILITY, ITS IMPORTANCE AND URGENT NEED TO INCREASE SOIL FERTILITY AND SUSTAINABLE CROP PRODUCTIVITY

Soil fertility is a vital aspect of agricultural ecosystems, influencing the soil's ability to supply essential nutrients crucial for optimal plant growth. This factor is pivotal for ensuring the success and sustainability of crop productivity.

The significance of soil fertility extends to the health of crops, the nutritional quality of harvested produce, and the overall resilience of agricultural systems. Recognizing the urgency to increase soil fertility has become a central concern for ensuring sustainable crop productivity and global food security. Soil fertility is synonymous with the soil's capacity to supply essential nutrients to plants. Key nutrients include nitrogen, phosphorus, potassium, sulfur, calcium, magnesium, and micronutrients like zinc and iron. Adequate nutrient levels are crucial for various physiological processes in plants, influencing their growth, flowering, fruiting, and overall productivity.

The nutritional composition of crops is directly affected by soil fertility. Nutrient-dense crops, vital for both human and animal health, flourish thanks to the nurturing embrace of well-fertilized soils. Inadequate soil fertility may result in nutrient deficiencies in crops, compromising their quality and nutritional value. Healthy soils support diverse microbial communities, including beneficial bacteria and fungi, contributing to nutrient cycling, disease suppression, and overall ecosystem resilience. This biodiversity enhances the stability and sustainability of agricultural ecosystems. Certain soil properties influenced by fertility, such as organic matter content, impact water retention and drainage. Well-structured, fertile soils can retain moisture for sustained periods, reducing the impact of drought stress on crops. Simultaneously, they facilitate proper drainage, preventing waterlogging, which can be detrimental to plant roots. Fertile soils contribute to climate change mitigation by enhancing carbon sequestration. Soils rich in organic matter store more carbon, playing a role in mitigating the effects of greenhouse gas emissions.

Embracing sustainable soil management techniques holds the key to not only sequestering carbon but also minimizing agriculture's carbon footprint. The urgency to increase soil fertility arises from the growing global population's demand for food production. To meet these demands sustainably, it is crucial to enhance soil fertility to ensure optimal crop yields and nutritional quality. Traditional agricultural practices, characterized by monoculture, excessive use of chemical fertilizers, and inadequate soil conservation measures, have led to soil degradation. Intensive farming has depleted soil fertility, necessitating urgent interventions to restore and maintain soil health. Soil erosion, loss of topsoil, and degradation of soil structure are prevalent issues associated with poor soil fertility. These environmental challenges contribute to reduced agricultural productivity and negatively impact water quality. Soil fertility is intricately linked to global food security. As arable land diminishes and climate change poses new challenges, optimizing the fertility of existing agricultural land becomes imperative to ensure a stable and secure food supply. Transitioning to sustainable agricultural practices is essential for increasing soil fertility. Innovative soil care embraces techniques like crop rotation, cover cropping, organic farming, and integrated nutrient management, nurturing soil health and ensuring sustained fertility over time (Figure 2.1).

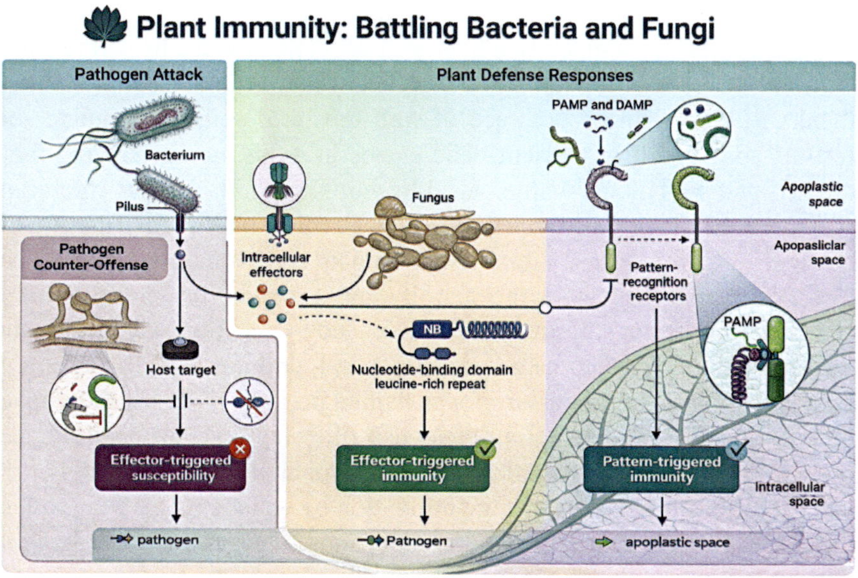

FIGURE 2.1 Evading the immune defenses of plants by microbial pathogens.

The continuous growth of the global population and increasing affluence are anticipated to intensify the demand for food in the coming years. According to estimates by the Food and Agriculture Organization (FAO), the world's population is expected to reach 9.6 billion by 2050. To meet this demand, food production must increase by 70%. This necessary increase in production is expected to be achieved on the same or slightly reduced arable land. However, water resources for crops will face heightened competition from industrial and other human needs. Moreover, the impending impacts of climate change, from shifts in crop life cycles and durations to heightened environmental strain, encompassing temperature fluctuations and water-related adversities like droughts and floods, will escalate.

2.2.1 UNDESIRABLE EFFECTS OF INCREASED INPUTS OF CHEMICAL FERTILIZERS AND PESTICIDES

The heightened crop productivity has alleviated the necessity of expanding cultivated areas, thereby preserving forests and indigenous vegetation along with their diverse biodiversity. Nevertheless, the drawbacks of employing advanced technologies involving elevated quantities of chemical fertilizers and pesticides manifested over subsequent years. These drawbacks encompass the emission of nitrogen oxides, identified as greenhouse gases, into the atmosphere, the runoff of nitrogen from fields leading to its accrual in aquatic ecosystems, and the degradation of soil coupled with the accumulation of pesticide residues. The development of resistance to pesticides in insect pests and pathogens, along with discernible impacts on human health, is now widely acknowledged, underscoring the additional concerns related to soil and groundwater contamination.

2.3 RHIZOSPHERE MICROBIAL DIVERSITY

The rhizosphere, characterized as the narrow soil zone profoundly influenced by the roots and root exudates of aboveground plants, stands as a hub of extensive microbial diversity. Comprising bacteria, actinomycetes, fungi, oomycetes, mycorrhiza, algae, protozoa, and nematodes, the rhizosphere has long been recognized as a crucial interface for plant-microbe interactions. Initial investigations into rhizosphere microbial populations were constrained to cultivable species, representing a mere fraction (less than 1%) of the actual microbial diversity. Advancements in molecular techniques, specifically those involving the isolation and characterization of nucleic acids from soil samples, have unveiled the existence of a staggering 6,000–10,000 different genomes per gram of soil (Torsvik et al., 1990).

Simultaneously, the repercussions of modern agricultural practices, marked by increased applications of chemical fertilizers and pesticides, have become apparent. These consequences encompass the release of nitrogen oxides, identified as greenhouse gases, into the atmosphere. Furthermore, there is the runoff of nitrogen from cultivated fields, contributing to its accumulation in water bodies, along with the degradation of soil and the buildup of pesticide residues. The emergence of pesticide resistance in insect pests and pathogens, coupled with the discernible impacts on human health, has become widely acknowledged, raising additional concerns related to soil and groundwater contamination.

The intricate dynamics of soil microbe and plant interactions add to the complexity of this ecosystem, dependent on numerous biological and environmental variables. Despite extensive research efforts, our understanding remains only partial (Reinhold-Hurek et al., 2015). The influence of soil microbes on plant growth can be either positive or negative. Positive impacts are exerted by biocontrol agents such as *Trichoderma* spp., *Bacillus subtilis*, and as well as plant growth promoters like PGPRs, rhizobia, mycorrhizae, free-living nitrogen fixers, and phosphate-solubilizing fungi and bacteria. Additionally, nonpathogenic strains of plant pathogens can outcompete their pathogenic counterparts, providing further positive contributions. Conversely, pathogens that overcome the natural defenses of crop plants elicit negative responses, resulting in reduced yields. Examples of such pathogens include *Fusarium* spp., *Rhizopus*, *Pythium*, *Ralstonia solanacearum*, and *Aspergilli* (Prasad et al., 2015). Classification of PGPRs is shown in Figure 2.2.

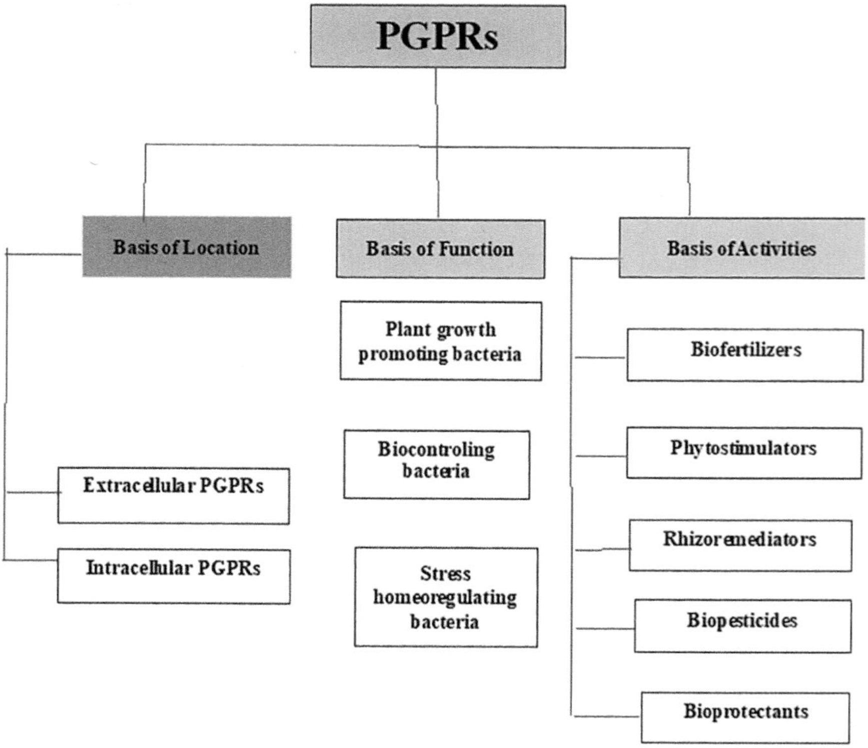

FIGURE 2.2 Classification of PGPRs.

Source: Adapted from Sharma et al. (2017).

2.3.1 ON THE BASIS OF LOCATION

As per the classification proposed by Gray and Smith (2005) and further expounded by Martinez-Viveros et al. (2010), PGPRs can be categorized into two distinct groups based on their localization within the rhizosphere. These groups are delineated as Extracellular PGPRs and Intracellular PGPRs.

2.3.2 EXTRACELLULAR PGPRS (EPGPRs)

These microorganisms inhabit the rhizosphere, reside on the rhizoplane, or occupy the intercellular spaces of the root cortex, refraining from penetrating the interior of the cells. Instances of such microorganisms include *Pseudomonas* and *Bacillus* species, which inhabit both the soil and the intercellular regions of cortical cells in an endophytic capacity.

2.3.3 INTRACELLULAR PGPRS (IPGPRs)

Typically, these microorganisms are predominantly found within cells, particularly within specialized nodular structures. Instances of such microorganisms include *Rhizobium* and *Frankia,* both of which form associations with higher plants and reside within the cells where they perform the crucial function of fixing atmospheric nitrogen.

2.3.4 ON THE BASIS OF FUNCTIONALITY

Based on this classification, PGPRs are categorized into three distinct groups: plant growth-promoting bacteria, biocontrol bacteria, and stress homeostasis-regulating bacteria.

2.4 PLANT GROWTH-PROMOTING BACTERIA

Specific rhizobacteria play an instrumental role in enhancing plant growth by directly engaging in mechanisms such as nitrogen fixation, synthesizing phytohormones like indole-3-acetic acid (IAA), cytokinin's, gibberellic acid (GA3), producing siderophores, and facilitating phosphate solubilization.

2.4.1 BIOCONTROLLING BACTERIA

Their contribution to plant growth extends beyond direct means; they indirectly foster growth by releasing compounds such as hydrogen cyanide, chitinase, pectinase, cellulase, ethylene, antibiotics, among others, with phytotoxic properties. These substances play a crucial role in managing plant pathogens and contribute to overall plant health.

2.4.2 STRESS HOMEOREGULATING BACTERIA

These versatile bacteria offer direct or indirect assistance to plant growth, adeptly navigating both biotic and abiotic stresses. Direct support includes the emission of stress-responsive phytohormones like abscisic acid, salicylic acid, and jasmonic acid, as well as plant growth regulators like cadaverine, and stress signaling molecules such as 1-aminocyclopropane-1-carboxylate (ACC) deaminase.

2.4.3 ON THE BASIS OF ACTIVITIES

On this basis, Somers et al. (2004) divide PGPRs into the following categories:

1. **Biofertilizers:** Many of the PGPRs contribute to soil fertility and productivity by participating in nutrient cycling. Various forms of biofertilizers are employed, including:

   i. Nitrogen-fixing biofertilizers like *Rhizobium, Bradyrhizobium, Nitrosomonas, Azospirillum, Azotobacter,* and so forth.
   ii. Phosphorus-solubilizing and phosphorus-mobilizing biofertilizers like *Bacillus, Pseudomonas, Mycorrhiza*, and so forth.
   iii. Plant growth-promoting biofertilizers like *Pseudomonas, Bacillus*, and so forth.

2. **Phytostimulators:** Certain bacteria stimulate plant growth by producing different phytohormones like *Pseudomonas, Azospirillum, Bradyrhizobium*, and so forth.

3. **Rhizoremediators:** Several bacteria are employed in the degradation of herbicides, pesticides, and other potentially harmful organic compounds or pollutants in the soil. This process can be beneficial for plant growth by enhancing soil fertility.

4. **Biopesticides:** Several bacteria have the capability to produce antibiotics and other toxic compounds, contributing to the suppression of pathogens. Examples of such bacteria include *Pseudomonas* and *Bacillus* species.

5. **Bioprotectants:** A multitude of bacteria play a crucial role in disease suppression, directly and indirectly contributing to the enhancement of plant growth.

2.4.4 USING PGPR FOR ENHANCED CROP PRODUCTION BY INCREASING SOIL FERTILITY

Plant growth-promoting rhizobacteria (PGPR) exhibit diverse traits that significantly contribute to the promotion and enhancement of plant growth. PGPRs employ an array of strategies to reshape the microbial community within the rhizosphere, thus nurturing plant growth across a spectrum of environmental conditions. Their facilitation of plant growth manifests through a blend of direct and indirect methodologies. Direct mechanisms involve nutrient supply, where PGPRs contribute essential elements like nitrogen, phosphorus, potassium, and minerals to plants. This is achieved through nitrogen fixation, mineral nutrient solubilization, mineralization of organic compounds, and the production of phytohormones. PGPRs play a crucial role in nitrogen fixation, offering a mutualistic relationship with plants. Symbiotic nitrogen fixation involves the formation of nodules in the roots, primarily with leguminous plants, where nitrogen is fixed and made available to the plant in the form of ammonia. *Rhizobia, including Rhizobium, Bradyrhizobium, Sinorhizobium,* and *Mesorhizobium,* engage in symbiotic interactions with leguminous plants, while *Frankia* associates with non-leguminous trees and shrubs. Non-symbiotic nitrogen fixation is facilitated by free-living diazotrophs, benefiting non-legume plants like radish and rice. Diazotrophic bacteria from various genera, such as *Azoarcus, Azotobacter, Acetobacter, Azospirillum, Burkholderia, Diazotrophicus, Enterobacter, Gluconacetobacter, Pseudomonas,* and *cyanobacteria* (*Anabaena, Nostoc*), actively participate in non-symbiotic nitrogen fixation. In the context of phosphorus availability, PGPRs employ strategies to make inaccessible forms of phosphorus available for plants. Key phosphate solubilization mechanisms include the production of organic acids, acid phosphatases, and siderophores. These mechanisms enhance the bioavailability of phosphorus in the rhizosphere, supporting plant growth. Indirect mechanisms of plant growth promotion by PGPRs involve the alleviation of inhibitory effects from various pathogens. PGPRs function as multifaceted allies, serving as biocontrol agents, root inhabitants, and guardians of the environment, effectively curbing the detrimental effects of pathogens on plant growth and development. The multifaceted contributions of PGPRs underscore their importance in sustainable agriculture, promoting plant health, and improving overall crop productivity. The liberation of compounds capable of complexing or dissolving minerals, such as organic acid anions, protons, hydroxyl ions, and CO_2, is a vital process for enhancing nutrient availability. Additionally, the secretion of extracellular enzymes, contributing to biochemical phosphate mineralization, plays a significant role in releasing phosphate from mineral compounds. Furthermore, the release of phosphate is facilitated during substrate degradation, a process known as biological phosphate mineralization.

2.5 ROLE OF PLANT GROWTH PROMOTING RHIZOBACTERIA AS A BIOFERTILIZER

Biofertilizers, dynamic in their essence, harbor living microorganisms that, when applied to seeds, plant surfaces, or soil, establish residence within the rhizosphere or the plant's interior. This colonization fosters plant growth by bolstering the supply or accessibility of primary nutrients to the host plant, as articulated by Vessey et al. (2003). Mishra et al. (2003) characterize biofertilizers as blends of active or dormant cells that promote nitrogen fixation, phosphate solubilization, or cellulose breakdown. These microorganisms enrich nutrient availability and find application in soil, seeds, roots, or composting areas, enriching the abundance of beneficial microorganisms. This amplifies microbial processes conducive to plants, facilitating nutrient assimilation and uptake. Proposing a definition, Malusà et al. (2014) denote biofertilizers as meticulously formulated products housing one or more microorganisms that enhance plant nutrient status, either by supplementing soil nutrients or rendering them more accessible to plants, thereby enhancing plant nutrient uptake. Typically, biofertilizer formulations are rooted in plant growth-promoting microorganisms (PGPM), which predominantly fall into three categories: Arbuscular mycorrhizal fungi (Jeffries et al., 2003), plant growth-promoting rhizobacteria (Podile et al., 2006), and nitrogen-fixing rhizobia (Franche et al., 2009).

PGPR, particularly strains of *Bacillus* spp. and *Pseudomonas* spp., have garnered widespread utilization as biofertilizers, augmenting crop productivity and soil fertility (Khalid et al., 2009). Studies conducted by Chen et al. (2011) propose that integrating PGPR with composts in biofertilizers amplifies growth-promoting properties and enhances plant biocontrol. Notably, *Bacillus* spp. and *Pseudomonas* spp. emerge as efficacious biocontrol agents, with *Bacillus subtilis*, *Bacillus amyloliquefaciens*, and *Bacillus cereus* demonstrating significant efficacy against plant pathogens (Francis et al., 2010). The ability of PGPR, especially *Bacillus* spp. and *Pseudomonas* spp., to form endospores equips them to endure diverse environmental conditions, facilitating the formulation of robust biofertilizers (Perez-Garcia et al., 2011).

Research by Waddington et al. (1998) underscores the pivotal role of optimal PGPR densities in biofertilizers in fostering a conducive rhizosphere for plant growth and mediating the transformation of essential nutrients via various biological processes. Yang et al. (2011) ascertains that high availability of nitrogen, phosphorus, and potassium bolsters soil fertility, enhances the biocontrol efficacy of antagonistic strains, and prolongs the survival of microorganisms in soil. When PGPR function as a source of plant nourishment and enrichment, facilitating the replenishment or restructuring of the nutrient cycle among soil, plant roots, and microorganisms, they qualify as biofertilizers. Nonetheless, the efficacy of "living" biofertilizers and the necessity for continual reapplication raise concerns regarding their self-sustainability and the potential disruption of microorganism interactions in soil with excessive usage.

2.5.1 CHALLENGES OF MICROBIAL PRODUCTION/PGPR PRODUCTION

The primary challenge hindering the widespread and efficient use of microbials lies in their nature as living entities, demanding meticulous attention in growth, formulation, delivery, and crop management practices. This necessitates education for manufacturers, dealers, and farmers to ensure proper handling. Unlike chemicals, the bioefficacy of microbials is often influenced by prevailing soil and crop health, diminishing farmers' confidence, especially among small and marginal farmers. Several strategies can enhance the bioefficacy of microbials, and one such approach involves combining them with a reduced dosage of chemicals, including fertilizers and pesticides. For successful integration, compatibility between biological and chemical components is crucial.

To modify the susceptibility of microbes to chemicals, induced mutagenesis can be employed. Despite successful research and development efforts, commercially available strains resulting from this approach are still lacking. Another challenge is the sustainability of efficacy over the entire crop duration, requiring repeated applications in many cases. This complicates their usage, particularly due to the absence of standardized package practices for microbials. Addressing these challenges is essential to foster greater confidence among farmers and promote the effective utilization of microbials in agricultural practices.

2.6 CONCLUSIONS AND OUTLOOK FOR THE FUTURE

In conclusion, the pivotal role of plant growth-promoting rhizobacteria (PGPR) in enhancing agricultural sustainability cannot be overstated. The intricate relationships between these beneficial microorganisms and plants have emerged as a promising avenue for promoting plant growth, ensuring food security, and mitigating the environmental impacts associated with traditional agricultural practices.

One of the pivotal roles of PGPR lies in its capacity to augment nutrient availability for plants. By means such as nitrogen fixation, phosphate solubilization, and the synthesis of growth-promoting compounds like phytohormones, PGPR directly modulate nutrient absorption and utilization by plants. This not only addresses soil nutrient scarcities but also diminishes dependence on synthetic fertilizers, thereby alleviating the environmental ramifications associated with their excessive application. Moreover, the multifaceted function of PGPR encompasses their ability for biocontrol. Serving as natural antagonists, these bacteria suppress deleterious pathogens, thus diminishing the necessity for chemical pesticides. This environmentally friendly approach not only safeguards crop vitality but also mitigates the ecological hazards linked to synthetic pesticide usage. The capacity of PGPR to elicit systemic resistance in plants further fortifies defense mechanisms against diseases, contributing to sustainable crop protection strategies. Agricultural sustainability is inherently linked to the conservation of soil health, and PGPR plays a crucial role in soil improvement. By enhancing soil structure, promoting aggregation, and contributing to the production of organic matter, PGPR fosters an environment conducive to plant growth. Additionally, their involvement in the degradation of organic pollutants and contaminants underscores their potential in soil remediation, contributing to the overall health of agroecosystems. PGPR's positive impact on water use efficiency is another facet of its role in agricultural sustainability. The ability to improve water absorption by host plant roots, modify crop physiology to reduce water stress responses, and explore soil profiles for essential minerals demonstrates the potential of PGPR in mitigating the challenges posed by water scarcity.

In regions grappling with water scarcity, the symbiosis between plants and PGPR holds promise as a means of conferring a survival advantage, rendering it an invaluable facet of sustainable agricultural methodologies. The burgeoning domain of induced resistance mediated by PGPR presents an intriguing avenue for sustainable agriculture. By priming the plant's intrinsic immune response, PGPR empower crops to withstand biotic stressors posed by diverse pathogens. This not only diminishes reliance on chemical fungicides but also bolsters the overall resilience of agroecosystems. Unraveling the intricacies of signaling pathways implicated in induced resistance paves the way for cultivating crops endowed with heightened natural defenses.

However, despite these promising attributes, the widespread adoption of PGPR encounters hurdles. The living nature of these microorganisms necessitates meticulous attention to cultivation, formulation, and application practices. Farmers, particularly smallholders, require education and awareness to harness the full potential of PGPR. Collaborative endeavors among researchers, manufacturers, and farmers are imperative for surmounting these obstacles and mainstreaming the integration of PGPR into agricultural practices.

In essence, plant growth-promoting rhizobacteria epitomize a sustainable and environmentally conscious approach to contemporary agriculture. Their diverse contributions, spanning nutrient regulation, biocontrol, soil vitality, and water conservation, position them as pivotal agents in the quest for agricultural sustainability. Amidst the complexities posed by a burgeoning global populace, environmental apprehensions, and the imperative to maximize yields with minimal resources, embracing the potential of PGPR emerges as a beacon illuminating the path towards a more sustainable and resilient agricultural future.

KEYWORDS

- **biological nitrogen fixation**
- **nutrient cycling**
- **phosphorus solubilization**
- **rhizosphere interactions**
- **soil fertility**
- **sustainable agriculture**

REFERENCES

Acosta-Durán, C., & Martínez-Romero, E. (2002). Diversity of rhizobia from nodules of the leguminous tree *Gliricidia sepium*, a natural host of *Rhizobium tropici*. *Archives of Microbiology*, *178*, 161–164.

Ahmad, F., Ahmad, I., & Khan, M. S. (2005). Indole acetic acid production by the indigenous isolates of *Azotobacter* and fluorescent *Pseudomonas* in the presence and absence of tryptophan. *Turkish Journal of Biology*, *29*, 29–34.

Ahmad, M., Zahir, Z. A., Khalid, M., et al. (2013). Efficacy of *Rhizobium* and *Pseudomonas* strains to improve physiology, ionic balance and quality of mung bean under salt-affected conditions on farmer's fields. *Plant Physiology and Biochemistry*, *63*, 170–176.

Ahmed, A., & Hasnain, S. (2010). Auxin producing *Bacillus* sp.: Auxin quantification and effect on the growth of *Solanum tuberosum*. *Pure and Applied Chemistry*, *82*, 313–319.

Aloni, R., Aloni, E., Langhans, M., et al. (2006). Role of cytokinin and auxin in shaping root architecture: Regulating vascular differentiation, lateral root initiation, root apical dominance and root gravitropism. *Annals of Botany*, *97*, 883–893.

Amarger, N. (2001). Rhizobia in the field. In *Advances in Agronomy*. London (UK): Academic Press.

Arora, N. K., Khare, E., Oh, J. H., et al. (2008). Diverse mechanisms adopted by *Pseudomonas fluorescens* PGC2 during the inhibition of *Rhizoctonia solani* and *Phytophthora capsici*. *World Journal of Microbiology and Biotechnology*, *24*, 581–585.

Basak, B. B., & Biswas, D. R. (2009). Influence of potassium solubilizing microorganism (*Bacillus mucilaginosus*) and waste mica on potassium uptake dynamics by sudan grass (*Sorghum vulgare* Pers.) grown under two Alfisols. *Plant and Soil*, *317*, 235–255.

Bedmar, E., Gonzálo, J., Lluch, C., et al. (2006). *Fijación de Nitrógeno: Fundamentos y Aplicaciones*. Granada: Sociedad Española de Microbiología (SEFIN).

Beneduzi, A., Ambrosini, A., & Passaglia, L. M. (2012). Plant growth-promoting rhizobacteria (PGPR): Their potential as antagonists and biocontrol agents. *Genetics and Molecular Biology*, *35*, 1044–1051.

Beneduzi, A., Peres, D., Vargas, L. K., Bodanese-Zanettini, M. H., & Passaglia, L. M. P. (2008). Evaluation of genetic diversity and plant growth promoting activities of nitrogen-fixing *Bacilli* isolated from rice fields in South Brazil. *Applied Soil Ecology, 39*, 311–320.

Bent, E., Tuzun, S., Chanway, C. P., et al. (2001). Alterations in plant growth and in root hormone levels of lodgepole pines inoculated with rhizobacteria. *Canadian Journal of Microbiology, 47*, 793–800.

Berg, G., & Smalla, K. (2009). Plant species and soil type cooperatively shape the structure and function of microbial communities in the rhizosphere. *FEMS Microbiology Ecology, 68*, 1–13. https://doi.org/10.1111/j.1574-6941.2009.00654.x (accessed on 2nd January 2026).

Berg, R. H., Tyler, M. E., Novick, N. J., et al. (1980). Biology of *Azospirillum*-sugarcane association: Enhancement of nitrogenase activity. *Applied and Environmental Microbiology, 39*, 642–649.

Bertrand, H., Nalin, R., Bally, R., & Cleyet-Marel, J. C. (2001). Isolation and identification of the most efficient plant growth-promoting bacteria associated with canola (*Brassica napus*). *Biology and Fertility of Soils, 33*, 152–156.

Bhatia, S., Dubey, R. C., & Maheshwari, D. K. (2005). Enhancement of plant growth and suppression of collar rot of sunflower caused by *Sclerotium rolfsii* through fluorescent *Pseudomonas*. *Indian Phytopathology, 58*, 17–24.

Biswas, J. C., Ladha, J. K., & Dazzo, F. B. (2000). Rhizobia inoculation improves nutrient uptake and growth of lowland rice. *Soil Science Society of America Journal, 64*, 1644–1650.

Cakmakci, R., Erat, M., Erdoğan, Ü. G., & Dönmez, M. F. (2007). The influence of PGPR on growth parameters, antioxidant and pentose phosphate oxidative cycle enzymes in wheat and spinach plants. *Journal of Plant Nutrition and Soil Science, 170*, 288–295.

Chandra, S., Choure, K., Dubey, R. C., & Maheshwari, D. K. (2007). Rhizosphere competent *Mesorhizobium loti* MP6 induces root hair curling, inhibits *Sclerotinia sclerotiorum* and enhances growth of Indian mustard (*Brassica campestris*). *Brazilian Journal of Microbiology, 38*, 124–130.

Chen, L. H., Tang, X. M., Raze, W., Li, J. H., Liu, Y. X., Qiu, M. H., Zhang, F. G., & Shen, Q. R. (2011). *Trichoderma harzianum* SQR-T037 rapidly degrades allelochemicals in rhizospheres of continuously cropped cucumbers. *Applied Microbiology and Biotechnology, 89*, 1653–1663.

De Felipe, M. R. (2006). Fijación biológica de dinitrógeno atmosférico en vidalibre. In Bedmar, E., Gonzálo, J., Lluch, C., et al. (Eds.), *Fijación de Nitrógeno: Fundamentos y Aplicaciones* (pp. 9–16). Granada: Sociedad Española de Microbiología (SEFIN).

De Freitas, J. R., Banerjee, M. R., & Germida, J. J. (1997). Phosphate-solubilizing rhizobacteria enhance the growth and yield but not phosphorus uptake of canola (*Brassica napus* L.). *Biology and Fertility of Soils, 24*, 358–364.

De Lajudie, P., Willems, A., Nick, G., et al. (1998). Characterization of tropical tree rhizobia and description of *Mesorhizobium plurifarium* sp. nov. *International Journal of Systematic Bacteriology, 48*, 369–382.

Dell'Amico, E., Cavalca, L., & Andreoni, V. (2008). Improvement of *Brassica napus* growth under cadmium stress by cadmium-resistant rhizobacteria. *Soil Biology and Biochemistry, 40*, 74–84.

Dey, R., Pal, K. K., Bhatt, D. M., & Chauhan, S. M. (2004). Growth promotion and yield enhancement of peanut (*Arachis hypogaea* L.) by application of plant growth promoting rhizobacteria. *Microbiological Research, 159*, 371–394.

Dobereiner, J. (1961). Nitrogen-fixing bacteria of the genus *Beijerinckia* Derx in the rhizosphere of sugar cane. *Plant and Soil, 15*, 211–216.

Egamberdieva, D. (2005). Plant growth promoting rhizobacteria isolated from a Calcisol in semi-arid region of Uzbekistan: Biochemical characterization and effectiveness. *Journal of Plant Nutrition and Soil Science, 168*, 94–99.

Egamberdiyeva, D. (2007). The effect of plant growth promoting bacteria on growth and nutrient uptake of maize in two different soils. *Applied Soil Ecology, 36*, 184–189.

El-Akhal, M. R., Rincon, A., Coba de la Peña, T., et al. (2013). Effects of salt stress and rhizobial inoculation on growth and nitrogen fixation of three peanut cultivars. *Plant Biology (Stuttgart), 15*, 415–421.

Elbeltagy, A., Nishioka, K., Sato, T., et al. (2001). Endophytic colonization and *in planta* nitrogen fixation by a *Herbaspirillum* sp. isolated from wild rice species. *Applied and Environmental Microbiology, 67*, 5285–5293.

Flores-Félix, J. D., Silva, L. R., Rivera, L. P., et al. (2015). Plants probiotics as a tool to produce highly functional fruits: The case of *Phyllobacterium* and vitamin C in strawberries. *PLoS ONE, 10*, e0122281. https://doi.org/10.1371/journal.pone.0122281 (accessed on 2nd January 2026).

Franche, C., Lindström, K., & Elmerich, C. (2009). Nitrogen-fixing bacteria associated with leguminous and non-leguminous plants. *Plant and Soil, 321*, 35–59.

Francis, I., Holsters, M., & Vereecke, D. (2010). The gram-positive side of plant-microbe interaction. *Environmental Microbiology, 12*, 1–12.

García de Salamone, I. E., Hynes, R. K., & Nelson, L. M. (2001). Cytokinin production by plant growth promoting rhizobacteria and selected mutants. *Canadian Journal of Microbiology, 47*, 404–411.

Glick, B. R. (1995). The enhancement of plant growth by free-living bacteria. *Canadian Journal of Microbiology, 41*, 109–117.

Gong, M., Wang, J. D., Zhang, J., & Yang, H. (2006). Study of the antifungal ability of *Bacillus subtilis* strain PY-1 *in vitro* and identification of its antifungal substance (Iturin A). *Acta Biochimica et Biophysica Sinica, 38*, 233–240.

Govindarajan, M., Balandreau, J., Kwon, S. W., et al. (2007). Effects of the inoculation of *Burkholderia vietnamensis* and related endophytic diazotrophic bacteria on grain yield of rice. *Microbial Ecology, 55*, 21–37.

Han, H. S., & Lee, K. D. (2005). Phosphate and potassium solubilizing bacteria effect on mineral uptake, soil availability and growth of eggplant. *Research Journal of Agriculture and Biological Sciences, 1*, 176–180.

Han, H. S., Supanjani, S., & Lee, K. D. (2006). Effect of co-inoculation with phosphate and potassium solubilizing bacteria on mineral uptake and growth of pepper and cucumber. *Plant, Soil and Environment, 52*, 130–136.

Hurek, T., & Reinhold-Hurek, B. (2003). *Azoarcus* sp. strain BH72 as a model for nitrogen-fixing grass endophytes. *Journal of Biotechnology, 106*, 169–178.

Jeffries, P., Gianinazzi, S., Perotto, S., Turnau, K., & Barea, J. M. (2003). The contribution of arbuscular mycorrhizal fungi in sustainable maintenance of plant health and soil fertility. *Biology and Fertility of Soils, 37*, 1–16.

Joo, G. J., Kim, Y. M., Kim, J. T., et al. (2005). Gibberellins-producing rhizobacteria increase endogenous gibberellins content and promote growth of red peppers. *Journal of Microbiology*, *43*, 510–515.

Kaneko, T., Nakamura, Y., Sato, S., et al. (2000). Complete genome structure of the nitrogen-fixing symbiotic bacterium *Mesorhizobium loti*. *DNA Research*, *7*, 331–338.

Kao, C. M., Chen, S. C., Chen, Y. S., et al. (2003). Detection of *Burkholderia pseudomallei* in rice fields with PCR-based technique. *Folia Microbiologica (Praha)*, *48*, 521–524.

Kaschuk, G., Hungria, M., Andrade, D. S., et al. (2006). Genetic diversity of rhizobia associated with common bean (*Phaseolus vulgaris* L.) grown under no-tillage and conventional systems in Southern Brazil. *Applied Soil Ecology*, *32*, 210–220.

Khalid, A., Arshad, M., Shaharoona, B., & Mahmood, T. (2009). Plant growth promoting rhizobacteria and sustainable agriculture. In *Microbial Strategies for Crop Improvement* (pp. 133–160). Springer: Berlin/Heidelberg, Germany.

Khan, A. L., Waqas, M., Kang, S. M., et al. (2014). Bacterial endophyte *Sphingomonas* sp. LK11 produces gibberellins and IAA and promotes tomato plant growth. *Journal of Microbiology*, *52*, 689–695.

Kumar, H., Bajpai, V. K., Dubey, R. C., et al. (2010). Wilt disease management and enhancement of growth and yield of *Cajanus cajan* (L.) var. Manak by bacterial combinations amended with chemical fertilizer. *Crop Protection*, *29*, 591–598.

Leonardo, D., Blanca, L. F., Landa, B., & Weller, D. M. (2006). Host crop affects rhizosphere colonization and competitiveness of 2,4-diacetylphloroglucinol producing *Pseudomonas fluorescens*. *Phytopathology*, *96*, 751–762.

Lindow, S. E., & Brandl, M. T. (2003). Microbiology of the phyllosphere. *Applied and Environmental Microbiology*, *69*, 1875–1883. https://doi.org/10.1128/aem.69.4.1875-1883.2003 (accessed on 2nd January 2026).

Liu, F., Xing, S., Ma, H., et al. (2013). Cytokinin-producing, plant growth-promoting rhizobacteria that confer resistance to drought stress in *Platycladus orientalis* container seedlings. *Applied Microbiology and Biotechnology*, *97*, 9155–9164.

Malusá, E., & Vassilev, N. A. (2014). Contribution to set a legal framework for biofertilizers. *Applied Microbiology and Biotechnology*, *98*, 6599–6607.

Mazzola, M., Fujimoto, D. K., Thomashow, L. S., et al. (1995). Variation in sensitivity of *Gaeumannomyces graminis* to antibiotics produced by fluorescent *Pseudomonas* spp. and effect on biological control of take-all of wheat. *Applied and Environmental Microbiology*, *61*, 2554–2559.

Mishra, D., Rajvir, S., Mishra, U., & Kumar, S. S. (2013). Role of biofertilizer in organic agriculture: A review. *Research Journal of Recent Sciences*, *2*, 39–41.

Muñoz-Rojas, J., & Caballero-Mellado, J. (2003). Population dynamics of *Gluconacetobacter diazotrophicus* in sugarcane cultivars and its effect on plant growth. *Microbial Ecology*, *46*, 454–464.

Muratova, A. Y., Turkovskaya, O. V., Antonyuk, L. P., Makarov, O. E., Pozdnyakova, L. I., & Ignatov, V. V. (2005). Oil-oxidizing potential of associative rhizobacteria of the genus *Azospirillum*. *Microbiology*, *74*, 210–215.

Patten, C. L., & Glick, B. R. (2002). Role of *Pseudomonas putida* indoleacetic acid in development of the host plant root system. *Applied and Environmental Microbiology*, *68*, 3795–3801.

Pereira, J. A. R., Cavalcante, V. A., Baldani, J. I., et al. (1988). Field inoculation of sorghum and rice with *Azospirillum* spp. and *Herbaspirillum seropedicae*. *Plant and Soil, 110*, 269–274.

Perez-Garcia, A., Romero, D., & de Vicente, A. (2011). Plant protection and growth stimulation by microorganism: Biotechnological applications of *Bacillus* in agriculture. *Current Opinion in Biotechnology*, *22*, 187–193.

Persello-Cartieaux, F., David, P., Sarrobert, C., Thibaud, M.-C., Achouak, W., Robaglia, C., & Nussaume, L. (2001). Utilization of mutants to analyze the interaction between *Arabidopsis thaliana* and its naturally root-associated *Pseudomonas*. *Planta, 212*, 190–198.

Pishchik, V. N., Vorobyev, N. I., Chernyaeva, I. I., Timofeeva, S. V., Kozhemyakov, A. P., Alexeev, Y. V., & Lukin, S. M. (2002). Experimental and mathematical simulation of plant growth promoting rhizobacteria and plant interaction under cadmium stress. *Plant and Soil*, *243*, 173–186.

Podile, A. R., & Kishore, G. K. (2006). Plant growth-promoting rhizobacteria. In *Plant-Associated Bacteria* (pp. 195–230). Springer: Dordrecht, the Netherlands.

Prasad, R., Kumar, M., & Varma, A. (2015). Role of PGPR in soil fertility and plant health. In Egamberdieva, D., Shrivastava, S., & Varma, A. (Eds.), *Plant Growth-Promoting Rhizobacteria (PGPR) and Medicinal Plants* (pp. 247–260). Springer International Publishing, Switzerland.

Radzki, W., Gutierrez Mañero, F. J., Algar, E., et al. (2013). Bacterial siderophores efficiently provide iron to iron-starved tomato plants in hydroponics culture. *Antonie van Leeuwenhoek*, *104*, 321–330.

Reinhold-Hurek, B., & Hurek, T. (1998). Interactions of gramineous plants with *Azoarcus* spp. and other diazotrophs: Identification, localization, and perspectives to study their function. *Critical Reviews in Plant Sciences*, *17*, 29–54.

Reinhold-Hurek, B., Bünger, W., Burbano, C. S., Sabale, M., & Hurek, T. (2015). Roots shaping their microbiome: Global hotspots for microbial activity. *Annual Review of Phytopathology*, *53*, 403–424.

Roesti, D., Guar, R., Johri, B. N., Imfeld, G., Sharma, S., Kawaljeet, K., & Aragno, M. (2006). Plant growth stage, fertilizer management and bio inoculation of arbuscular mycorrhizal fungi and plant growth promoting rhizobacteria affect the rhizobacterial community structure in rain-fed wheat field. *Soil Biology and Biochemistry*, *38*, 1111–1120.

Sabry, S. R. S., Saleh, S. A., Batchelor, C. A., et al. (1997). Endophytic establishment of *Azorhizobium caulinodans* in wheat. *Proceedings of the Biological Sciences*, *264*, 341–346.

Sahoo, R. K., Ansari, M. W., Pradhan, M., et al. (2014). Phenotypic and molecular characterization of native *Azospirillum* strains from rice fields to improve crop productivity. *Protoplasm*, *251*, 943–953.

Sangeeth, K. P., Bhai, R. S., & Srinivasan, V. (2012). *Paenibacillus glucanolyticus*, a promising potassium solubilizing bacterium isolated from black pepper (*Piper nigrum* L.) rhizosphere. *Journal of Spices and Aromatic Crops*, *21*, 118–124.

Shaharoona, B., Naveed, M., Arshad, M., et al. (2008). Fertilizer-dependent efficiency of *Pseudomonas* for improving growth, yield, and nutrient use efficiency of wheat (*Triticum aestivum* L.). *Applied Microbiology and Biotechnology*, *79*, 147–155.

Sheng, X. F., & He, L. Y. (2006). Solubilization of potassium-bearing minerals by a wild-type strain of *Bacillus edaphicus* and its mutants and increased potassium uptake by wheat. *Canadian Journal of Microbiology*, *52*, 66–72.

Silo-Suh, L. A., Lethbridge, B. J., Raffel, S. J., et al. (1994). Biological activities of two fungistatic antibiotics produced by *Bacillus cereus* UW85. *Applied and Environmental Microbiology*, *60*, 2023–2030.

Simonet, P., Normand, P., Moiroud, A., et al. (1990). Identification of *Frankia* strains in nodules by hybridization of polymerase chain reaction products with strain-specific oligonucleotide probes. *Archives of Microbiology*, *153*, 235–240.

Sokolova, M. G., Akimova, G. P., & Vaishlia, O. B. (2011). Effect of phytohormones synthesized by rhizosphere bacteria on plants. *Prikladnaya Biokhimiya i Mikrobiologiya*, *47*, 302–307.

Tejera, N., Lluch, C., Martínez-Toledo, M. V., et al. (2005). Isolation and characterization of *Azotobacter* and *Azospirillum* strains from the sugarcane rhizosphere. *Plant and Soil*, *270*, 223–232.

Thakuria, D., Taleekdar, N. C., Goswami, C., Hazarika, S., Boro, R. C., & Khan, M. R. (2004). Characterization and screening of bacteria from rhizosphere of rice grown in acidic soils of Assam. *Current Science*, *86*, 978–985.

Thamer, S., Schädler, M., Bonte, D., et al. (2011). Dual benefit from a belowground symbiosis: Nitrogen-fixing rhizobia promote growth and defense against a specialist herbivore in a cyanogenic plant. *Plant and Soil*, *341*, 209–219.

Timms-Wilson, T. M., Smalla, K., Goodall, T. I., Houlden, A., Gallego, V., et al. (2006). Microbial diversity in the phyllosphere and rhizosphere of field-grown crop plants: Microbial specialization at the plant surface. In Bailey, M. J., Lilley, A. K., & Timms-Wilson, T. M. (Eds.), *Microbial Ecology of Aerial Plant Surfaces* (pp. 21–36). CAB International: Wallingford.

Torsvik, V., Salte, K., Sørheim, R., & Goksøyr, J. (1990). Comparison of phenotypic diversity and DNA heterogeneity in a population of soil bacteria. *Applied and Environmental Microbiology*, *56*, 776–783.

Verma, V. C., Singh, S. K., & Prakash, S. (2011). Bio-control and plant growth promotion potential of siderophore-producing endophytic *Streptomyces* from *Azadirachta indica* A. Juss. *Journal of Basic Microbiology*, *51*, 550–556.

Vessey, J. K. (2003). Plant growth-promoting rhizobacteria as biofertilizers. *Plant and Soil*, *255*, 571–586.

Waddington, S. R. (1998). Organic matter management: From science to practice. *Soil Fertility*, *62*, 24–25.

Wani, S. A., Chand, S., & Ali, T. (2013). Potential use of *Azotobacter chroococcum* in crop production: An overview. *Current Agriculture Research Journal*, *1*, 35–38.

Wei, H. G., Tan, Z. Y., Zhu, M. E., et al. (2003). Characterization of rhizobia isolated from legume species within the genera *Astragalus* and *Lespedeza* grown in the Loess Plateau of China and description of *Rhizobium loessense* sp. nov. *International Journal of Systematic and Evolutionary Microbiology*, *53*, 1575–1583.

Yang, C. H., Crowley, D. E., Borneman, J., & Keen, N. T. (2001). Microbial phyllosphere populations are more complex than previously realized. *Proceedings of the National Academy of Sciences of the United States of America*, *98*, 3889–3894. https://doi.org/10.1073/pnas.051633898 (accessed on 2nd January 2026).

Yang, X., Chen, L., Yong, X., & Shen, Q. (2011). Formulations can affect rhizosphere colonization and biocontrol efficiency of *Trichoderma harzianum* SQR-T037 against *Fusarium* wilt of cucumbers. *Biology and Fertility of Soils, 47*, 239–248.

Yanni, Y., Rizk, R., Abd-El Fattah, F., et al. (2001). The beneficial plant growth-promoting association of *Rhizobium leguminosarum* bv. *trifolii* with rice roots. *Australian Journal of Plant Physiology, 28*, 845–870.

Yao, L., Wu, Z., Zheng, Y., et al. (2010). Growth promotion and protection against salt stress by *Pseudomonas putida* Rs-198 on cotton. *European Journal of Soil Biology, 46*, 49–54.

Yao, Z. Y., Kan, F. L., Wang, E. T., et al. (2002). Characterization of rhizobia that nodulate legume species of the genus *Lespedeza* and description of *Bradyrhizobium yuanmingense* sp. nov. *International Journal of Systematic and Evolutionary Microbiology, 52*, 2219–2230.

Young, J. P. W., & Haukka, K. E. (1996). Diversity and phylogeny of rhizobia. *New Phytologist, 133*, 87–94.

Zahir, Z. A., Abbas, S. A., Khalid, M., & Arshad, M. (2000). Substrate-dependent microbially derived plant hormones for improving growth of maize seedlings. *Pakistan Journal of Biological Sciences, 3*, 289–291.

CHAPTER 3

Phosphate-Solubilizing Bacteria: Role in Sustainable Agriculture

PRITI PAL,[1] AKHILESH KUMAR SINGH,[2] MAHARUDRA PRATAP SINGH,[2] UTTAM KUMAR SAHOO,[3] ANAND PRAKASH,[2] BRIJESH PANDEY,[2] RISHI KUMAR SINGH,[4] and PRAKASH KUMAR SARANGI[5,*]

[1]*Amity Institute of Biotechnology, Amity University Uttar Pradesh, Lucknow Campus, Lucknow, India*

[2]*Department of Biotechnology, School of Life Sciences, Mahatma Gandhi Central University, Motihari, Bihar, India*

[3]*Department of Forestry, Mizoram University, Aizawl, Mizoram, India*

[4]*School of Biosciences, IMS Institute, University Courses Campus, Ghaziabad, Uttar Pradesh, India*

[5]*College of Agriculture, Central Agricultural University, Imphal, Manipur, India*

*Corresponding authors

ABSTRACT

Soil microorganisms serve as custodians of ecological balance, dynamically participating in the carbon, nitrogen, sulfur, and phosphorus cycles within nature's intricate web. Phosphate-solubilizing microbes hold particular significance in enhancing plant nutrition by augmenting phosphate uptake and serving as biofertilizers for agricultural crops. Phosphorus, a crucial macronutrient for plant growth and development, is often limited in its availability in soils due to fixation as insoluble phosphates of iron,

Biotechnology for Sustainable Agriculture: Innovative Approaches and Strategies.
Prakash Kumar Sarangi (Ed)

DOI: 10.1201/9781779642998-3

aluminum, and calcium. Given the low availability of phosphorus in soils, attributed to its fixation as insoluble phosphates, chemical phosphatic fertilizers are extensively employed to achieve optimal yields. However, the drawback lies in the susceptibility of soluble forms of phosphatic fertilizers to precipitation as insoluble forms, necessitating excessive and recurrent applications. Phosphorus stands as a critical element for the functionality of key enzymes regulating metabolic pathways crucial for plant growth. Phosphorus exists in various forms in the soil solution, with roots absorbing different forms, predominantly $H_2PO_4^-$ and HPO_4^{2-} contingent upon soil pH. The sequestration and precipitation of phosphorus within soil are intricately governed by variables such as pH levels, moisture content, temperature fluctuations, and the prevailing mineral composition of the soil matrix.

3.1 INTRODUCTION

Minerals, organic constituents, and microorganisms constitute the three primary solid components of soil, exerting substantial influence on terrestrial systems and influencing physical, chemical, and biological properties. Soil infertility stands as a critical constraint, particularly impeding crop yields in developing nations, especially among impoverished farmers. Concurrently, the prolonged use of chemical fertilizers detrimentally impacts the health of indigenous soil microorganisms, altering soil pH levels. This acidity modification diminishes the presence of beneficial microorganisms crucial for enhancing plant and soil health, reinforcing plants' natural defenses against pests and diseases. Maintaining soil integrity stands as a paramount concern for agricultural practitioners, with the rejuvenation of soil fertility achievable through the implementation of integrated soil fertility management (ISFM). This holistic approach harmonizes tactics for biological nitrogen fixation (BNF) alongside initiatives aimed at optimizing input efficacy, as highlighted by Vlek and Vielhauer (1994). Biofertilizers play a vital role in integrated nutrient management, serving as products containing cells of diverse beneficial microorganisms. In this scenario, microorganisms assume a leading role in directing the intricate processes that regulate the conversion and availability of soil phosphorus to plants. Numerous soil microorganisms demonstrate the capability to solubilize or mineralize insoluble soil phosphate, releasing soluble phosphorus for plant utilization, thereby enhancing the growth and yield of various crops.

Commonly employed biofertilizer components include nitrogen-fixing organisms (N-fixers), potassium-solubilizing organisms (K-solubilizers), phosphorus-solubilizing organisms (P-solubilizers), often in combination with molds or fungi. The utilization of microorganisms and reduced reliance on conventional phosphorus fertilizers as inoculants to mobilize less available phosphorus sources in the soil presents a promising alternative. This methodology not only curbs environmental degradation but also amplifies crop output to fulfill the surging global food requisites. It tackles apprehensions associated with surface and groundwater contamination, waterway eutrophication, soil fertility degradation, and the buildup of hazardous elements such as selenium (Se) and arsenic (As) in the soil. Within this framework, beneficial microorganisms, including antibiotic-generating bacteria and various fungi like mycorrhizal, thrive within vibrant soil ecosystems. Thus, inoculating seeds, crops, or soil with Phosphate Solubilizing Microorganisms (PSM) emerges as a promising strategy to elevate global food production without posing environmental hazards. While laboratory, greenhouse, and open field trials affirm the clear benefits of these technologies in improving soil fertility, phosphorus-solubilizing microorganisms have not yet supplanted conventional chemical fertilizers in commercial agriculture. The employment of phosphate-solubilizing bacteria (PSB) as inoculants presents a twofold advantage by amplifying plant phosphorus absorption and augmenting crop productivity. Notably, strains hailing from the genera *Pseudomonas, Bacillus,* and *Rhizobium* stand out for their potent phosphate-solubilizing prowess. The principal mechanism driving mineral phosphate solubilization revolves around the secretion of organic acids, with acid phosphatases assuming a pivotal role in the mineralization of organic phosphorus in soil. Genetic manipulation of PSB holds promise for bolstering their plant growth-promoting capabilities. This entails genetic engineering techniques like cloning and expression of genes associated with both mineral and organic phosphate solubilization, potentially introducing them into selected rhizobacterial strains under suitable promoters, as elucidated by Deubel and Merbach (2005).

Phosphorus serves as an integral component in various biological molecules, including nucleic acids, phospholipids, phytin, co-enzymes, phosphorylated sugars, and nucleotides. Highlighted by Sanyal and De Datta (1991) and further expounded upon by Kapoor (1995), this element assumes a pivotal function in fundamental cellular activities encompassing cell division, photosynthesis, carbohydrate metabolism, energy transference, and nutrient absorption. The fixation of phosphorus in soil has been estimated to be approximately 75% of the applied content. Notably, certain soil microorganisms, including bacteria and fungi, play a central role in the natural phosphorus cycle, facilitating the hydrolysis of phosphorus into its inorganic form, thereby enhancing its availability to plants. These enzymatic processes are mediated by phosphatase enzymes, as elucidated by Sobral (2003). Ensuring an ample supply of phosphorus during the early stages of plant growth holds paramount importance, particularly in the development of primordia for the reproductive parts of plants, as emphasized by Gaur (1990). The high-energy phosphate bonds associated with phosphorus play vital roles in respiratory and photosynthetic processes. Deficiency in this essential mineral nutrient manifests as stunted plant growth, characterized by deep green coloration, tilted petioles and leaflets, crinkly foliage, and the abnormal expansion failure of leaflets, as highlighted by Gaur (1990) and Sharma and Parmar (1997).

3.2 IMPORTANCE OF PHOSPHORUS SOLUBILIZING MICROORGANISMS

Organic acid production stands as a pivotal mechanism in the mineralization of phosphates in soil, primarily facilitated by the microbial secretion of low molecular weight organic acids. PSB exhibit the capability to lower the pH of their surroundings through the production of organic acids (Chen et al., 2006). These organic acids play a dual role—they can either dissolve phosphates via anion exchange or form chelates with Ca, Fe, or Al ions associated with phosphates (Gyaneshwar et al., 2002). However, the capacity of soil microorganisms to secrete organic acids and, consequently, solubilize mineral phosphates varies significantly among different species. Another crucial aspect involves the production of acid phosphatase, a process fundamental to the mineralization of phosphorus compounds. Numerous phosphatases, also known as phosphor hydrolases, are present in a diverse array of soil microorganisms and play a vital role in facilitating the assimilation of phosphate from organic compounds by both plants and microorganisms (Sharma et al., 2013). This process involves the hydrolysis of phosphoester or phosphor anhydride bonds. The impact of PSB on crop production is substantial, with the potential to increase crop yields by up to 70% (Mohammadi, 2011). The use of phosphate-solubilizing microorganisms (PSMs) as inoculants concurrently enhances plant phosphorus uptake and crop yield. Strains of PSB exhibiting multiple plant growth-promoting traits in the soil-plant system require further exploration to unveil their efficacy as bio-inoculants. Combining the inoculation of PSB with plant growth-promoting rhizobacteria (PGPR) has shown promise, reducing P fertilizer application by 50% without a significant decrease in crop yield (Sharma et al., 2011). Several soil bacteria, particularly those belonging to *Bacillus* and *Pseudomonas* genera, alongside fungi such as *Penicillium* and *Aspergillus,* exhibit the capability to convert insoluble phosphates in soil into soluble forms by exuding a spectrum of organic acids including formic, acetic, propionic, lactic, glycolic, fumaric, and succinic acids (Rashid et al., 2004). For instance, findings from Poonguzhali et al. (2008) underscored the significant enhancement in root length and biomass of Chinese cabbage (*Brassica rapa*) by phosphate-solubilizing strains of *Pseudomonas*. These strains, producing indole-3-acetic acid (IAA), 1-aminocyclopropane-1-carboxylate (ACC) deaminase, and siderophores, exhibited notable growth-promoting effects without compromising phosphorus uptake, hinting at mechanisms beyond phosphate solubilization. Combined inoculation of arbuscular mycorrhiza and PSBs has been shown to enhance plant growth through improved uptake of both native soil phosphorus and phosphorus derived from phosphatic rock fractions (Ahmed et al., 2008).

PSBs demonstrate the capacity to synthesize phytohormones such as Indole acetic acid (IAA), Gibberellic acid (GA3), and siderophores (Babna et al., 2013; Ramkumar and Kannapiran, 2011). Moreover, PSBs contribute to augmented plant growth by enhancing the efficiency of BNF and elevating the availability of trace elements like iron and zinc (Ponmurugan and Gopi, 2006). Studies have reported positive impacts on the growth and yield of various crops, including *Zea mays* (Yasmin et al., 2012) and wheat (Afzal et al., 2005). Additionally, the combined application of PSB and NPK has been found to positively influence the germination and seed quality of plants like radish, directly improving the vigor index (Lamo et al., 2012).

3.3 PHOSPHATE SOLUBILIZING BACTERIA

PSB represent advantageous microorganisms with the capability to solubilize fixed phosphorus in the soil. This process involves the conversion of the inorganic, unavailable phosphorus forms to soluble forms, namely $H_2PO_4^-$ and $H_2PO_4^-$, facilitated by organic acid production, chelation, and ion exchange reactions. Bacteria exhibit higher efficacy in phosphorus solubilization compared to fungi, as noted by Alam et al. (2002). PSB, functioning as an alternative to chemical fertilizers, demonstrate proficiency in phosphorous solubilization, production of plant growth hormones, and biocontrol activities. These free-living soil bacteria, predominantly isolated from the rhizosphere, exert their beneficial effects when applied as seed or crop inoculants. Their impact on plant growth and yield is achieved through various mechanisms, including the creation of phytohormones, provision of available nitrogen via BNF, solubilization of available phosphorus, and the suppression of diseases through phytohormones. Despite their relatively low P solubilization potential, ranging from 0.1% to 0.5%, in comparison to chemical fertilizers (Chen et al., 2006), the use of PSB in agriculture serves to offset the high costs associated with manufacturing phosphate fertilizers. Moreover, they mobilize insoluble phosphates in both fertilizers and soils, offering a sustainable and environmentally friendly solution for farmers (Banerjee et al., 2010; Chang and Yang, 2009).

Positioned as phosphate biofertilizers, PSBs play a crucial role in addressing the nutritional needs of plants, especially regarding phosphorus (P), a vital macronutrient. Traditionally, P is applied to soil in the form of phosphate fertilizers; however, a significant portion of the applied soluble inorganic phosphate rapidly immobilizes and becomes inaccessible to plants. Researchers routinely isolate and screen PSBs using Pikovskaya's (PVK) medium, with the solubilization of inorganic phosphate primarily attributed to the secretion of organic acids. Although the efficiency of isolates is often assessed by the formation of visible zones on Pikovskaya's agar medium plates containing tricalcium phosphate (TCP), it is important to note that certain isolates may not exhibit visible zones but can effectively solubilize various types of insoluble inorganic phosphates in a liquid medium.

Noteworthy bacterial genera, including *Azotobacter, Bacillus, Beijerinckia, Burkholderia, Enterobacter, Erwinia, Flavobacterium, Microbacterium, Pseudomonas, Rhizobium,* and *Serratia,* are recognized as highly significant PSB (Bhattacharyya et al., 2012). Their role in enhancing nutrient availability and promoting sustainable agriculture positions them as valuable contributors to soil health and plant productivity.

3.4 OCCURRENCE OF PHOSPHATE SOLUBILIZING BACTERIA

A significant portion of phosphate-solubilizing microorganisms (PSMs) congregates within the rhizosphere, showcasing heightened metabolic activity compared to other sources. Within soil, prevalent PSM examples encompass species of *Pseudomonas, Bacillus, Micrococcus, Flavobacterium, Aspergillus, Penicillium, Fusarium,* and *Sclerotium*. Particularly, strains from bacterial genera like *Pseudomonas, Bacillus, Rhizobium,* and *Enterobacter*, in addition to *Penicillium* and *Aspergillus* fungi, emerge as potent phosphate solubilizers. These microorganisms also extend their presence to rhizoplane soils. In terms of morphology, soil bacteria manifest diverse shapes such as cocci, bacilli, or spiral forms, with bacilli being predominant and *spirilla* being less common in natural habitats. The population density of PSB is contingent upon various soil attributes, including physical and chemical characteristics, organic matter content, phosphorus levels, and anthropogenic activities. Agricultural lands often harbor substantial populations of PSB. Optimal phosphorus (P) availability is typically observed within a pH range of 5.5 to 7, where P fixation occurs via hydrous oxides of Fe, Al, and Mn. Additionally, P fixation takes place through silicate minerals within pH 6 to 8 and via Ca within pH 6.5 to 8.5. Swaby and Sperber (1958) observed a higher population of phosphate-solubilizing microorganisms (20–40% of the total population) in the rhizosphere compared to the non-rhizosphere (10–15% of the total population). Reyes and Valduz (2006) explored the biodiversity of PSM in rhizospheric and bulk soils of colonizer plants at an abandoned rock phosphate mine, revealing a greater abundance of PSM in the rhizosphere than in bulk soil. Microbial diversity investigations by Neal et al. (1973) in wheat cultivars indicated higher populations of various microbes, including total bacteria, cellulolytic, pectinolytic, amylolytic, ammonifying, and nitrate-reducing microbes, in rhizospheric soil compared to non-rhizospheric soil. Optimal utilization of P in neutral and calcareous soils occurs within a pH range of 6 to 7 (Sharpley, 2006). Microorganisms involved in phosphorus acquisition include mycorrhizal fungi and PSMs (Fankem et al., 2006). Within soil bacterial communities, ectorhizosphere strains from *Pseudomonas* and *Bacilli,* as well as endosymbiotic rhizobia, have been identified as effective phosphate solubilizers (Whitelaw et al., 2000). Specific strains such as *Bacillus megaterium, B. circulans, B. subtilis, B. polymyxa, B. sircalmous, Pseudomonas striata*, and *Enterobacter,* are underscored as crucial contributors to phosphate solubilization (Kucey et al., 1989). Additionally, the nematophagous fungus *Arthrobotrys oligospora* exhibits proficiency in solubilizing phosphate rocks (Duponnois et al., 2006).

3.4.1 PHYTOHORMONES

Phytohormones function as vital chemical messengers responsible for orchestrating the growth and maturation of plants, exerting a profound influence on plant development by modulating the synthesis of hormones and other compounds crucial for plant growth. Among these, auxins, a prominent class of phytohormones, play a pivotal role in fostering lateral root formation, thereby enhancing the plant's capacity for nutrient absorption. Additionally, various other classes of plant hormones, including gibberellins, cytokinin's, ethylene, and abscisic acid, intricately regulate plant structure and influence processes such as seed germination, flowering time, sex determination in flowers, leaf aging, and fruit maturation. These phytohormones exert their effects through regulating gene expression, transcriptional activity, cell division, and growth, thereby governing crucial aspects of plant development such as pattern formation, vegetative and reproductive growth, and responses to environmental stresses.

Key plant processes, including leaf and flower initiation, fruit development, and ripening, are finely tuned and controlled by hormonal actions. In response to growth-limiting environmental conditions, plants often adjust the levels of their endogenous phytohormones as an adaptive strategy to mitigate stress effects. While this inherent response mechanism can be effective, rhizosphere microorganisms may also contribute to the modulation or production of phytohormones under controlled laboratory conditions. Consequently, numerous Plant Growth-Promoting Bacteria (PGPB) possess the capability to manipulate phytohormone levels, thereby influencing the hormonal equilibrium of plants and their response to stress factors.

Among the phytohormones synthesized, indole-3-acetic acid (IAA), an auxin known for its pivotal role in root development and cell division stimulation, stands out. Various bacteria, including *Aeromonas verona*, *Agrobacterium* sp., *Azospirillum brasiliense*, *Bradyrhizobium* sp., *Rhizobium* sp., and *Enterobacter* sp., are recognized producers of this hormone. As emphasized by Mirza et al. (2001), the intricate interplay between plants and microorganisms involves the dynamic modulation of phytohormone levels, ultimately contributing to the overall growth and stress response of plants.

3.4.2 INDOLE ACETIC ACID (IAA)

Indole-3-acetic acid (IAA), a pivotal auxin, assumes a critical role in orchestrating diverse morphological and physiological functions in plants, including cell expansion, division, tissue specialization, and responses to environmental cues like light and gravity. The synthesis of IAA, reliant on L-tryptophan as a precursor, profoundly influences plant development. Bacterial IAA producers (BIPs) possess the capacity to influence these processes by contributing IAA to the plant's auxin reservoir, with resultant effects contingent upon the amount of IAA produced. Notably, plant organs, particularly roots, exhibit heightened sensitivity to fluctuations in IAA levels. Elevated exogenous IAA prompts primary root elongation, as well as the formation of lateral and adventitious roots (Finnie and Van Staden, 1985). It is worth noting that IAA biosynthesis extends beyond higher plants; bacteria, fungi, and algae can also synthesize physiologically active IAA, which profoundly impacts plant growth and development. Numerous bacteria from the rhizosphere showcase the ability to synthesize IAA under controlled conditions, with or without physiological precursors such as tryptophan (Trp) (Caron et al., 1995; Davies, 1995; Glick, 2012). While IAA is implicated in various physiological processes such as root growth stimulation, salt stress alleviation, plant-pathogen interactions, legume-rhizobia interactions, and induction of systemic resistance against diseases, its primary role lies in fostering lateral root proliferation. This process increases root surface area, thereby enhancing water and nutrient absorption by the plant. Several PSB in soils have been observed to release IAA, which is subsequently absorbed by plant roots, augmenting the endogenous pool of plant IAA (Glick et al., 2007). However, the effects of varying IAA concentrations differ among different plant species. Optimal concentrations of bacterial IAA stimulate root growth, while high concentrations inhibit it (Glick, 2012). In metal-contaminated environments, bacterial IAA aids host plants in adapting to metal stress by eliciting physiological alterations in plant cell metabolism. This adaptive mechanism enables plants to tolerate high concentrations of heavy metals (Glick, 2010). However, Hao et al. (2012) demonstrated, through transposon mutagenesis in phosphate-solubilizing *Agrobacterium tumefaciens* CCNWGS0286, that bacterial IAA had a more significant impact on the growth of host plants under metal stress compared to bacterial metal resistance.

3.4.3 ETHYLENE LEVELS

At low concentrations, it has been observed that ethylene promotes plant growth. However, at moderate to high levels, it may impede root elongation. In plants, the conversion of ACC and 5'-deoxy-5'methylthioadenosine (MTA) to ACC is catalyzed by ACC synthase. Numerous plant growth-promoting bacteria have been identified to harbor the enzyme ACC deaminase. This enzyme functions by cleaving and sequestering the plant ethylene precursor ACC, consequently reducing the overall level of ethylene in a developing or stressed plant. The presence of these plant growth-promoting bacteria serves to modulate the concentration of ACC, preventing it from reaching levels where it may adversely affect root growth.

3.4.4 SIDEROPHORE PRODUCTION

PSB play a crucial role in the provision of phosphorus to plants and contribute to enhanced plant growth through various plant growth promotion activities, such as the production of siderophores. Siderophores are extracellular metabolites known to increase the availability of iron while concurrently suppressing the growth of soil-borne plant pathogens. The significance of siderophores produced by specific genera of Plant Growth-Promoting Rhizobacteria (PGPR) in plant growth promotion was first reported by Kloepper et al. (1980). Siderophores, often described as microbial Fe-chelating low molecular weight compounds, serve as essential contributors to the plant growth process. The presence of siderophore-producing PGPR in the rhizosphere enhances the supply of Fe^{3+} to plants, thereby fostering increased plant growth and crop productivity. Additionally, after chelating Fe^{3+}, these compounds create a Fe^{3+} deficient environment in the soil for other soil microbes. Consequently, this inhibits the activity of competitive microbes in the soil, further supporting the positive impact of PSB on plant growth.

3.4.5 NITROGEN FIXATION

The availability of nitrogen has emerged as a critical factor limiting plant growth due to factors such as rainfall and mineral leaching into groundwater. Several bacteria possess the capability to fix atmospheric nitrogen (N_2) and enhance its accessibility to plants. While PSB demonstrate nitrogen-fixing abilities, their contribution may not suffice to meet the plants' nitrogen requirements adequately. However, these bacteria, through their impact on shoot elongation and stimulation of nitrate (NO_3^-) transport systems, significantly augment the plants' nitrogen uptake. Despite not independently fixing a substantial amount of nitrogen for plant sustenance, their influence leads to an increased intake of nitrogen by the plants (Figure 3.1).

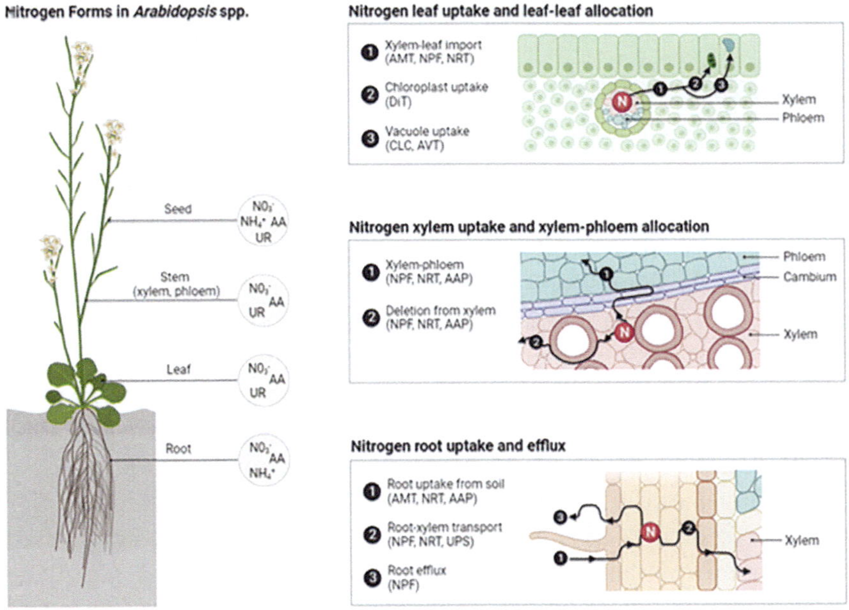

FIGURE 3.1 Nitrogen absorption and allocation.

3.5 INDUCED SYSTEMIC RESISTANCE

IAA production stands as a prominent attribute of rhizosphere bacteria, contributing to the stimulation and facilitation of plant growth. PSB and plant growth-promoting bacteria (PGPB) exhibit the ability to regulate the population of pathogenic bacteria through microbial antagonism. This antagonistic relationship is achieved by engaging in competition with pathogens for nutrients, synthesizing antibiotics, and producing antifungal metabolites. Apart from microbial antagonism, specific interplays between bacteria and plants trigger mechanisms that bolster the plant's immunity against pathogenic bacteria, fungi, and viruses. This phenomenon, known as induced systemic resistance (ISR), was initially expounded upon by Van Peer et al. (1991). The rhizobacteria inducing ISR initiate a response in the roots, generating a signal that diffuses throughout the entire plant. This activation leads to the reinforcement of the plant cell wall, the production of antimicrobial phytoalexins, and the synthesis of pathogen-related proteins as part of the plant's defense mechanisms. Components of bacteria that can activate ISR include lipopolysaccharides (LPS), flagella, salicylic acid, and siderophores.

3.5.1 BIOFERTILIZER

In agricultural contexts, beneficial bacteria find utility as inoculants for crops and plants, earning the designation of biofertilizer. Biofertilizers encompass substances containing living microorganisms that, upon application to seeds, plant surfaces, or soil, foster growth by amplifying the supply or accessibility of primary nutrients to the host plant. It is crucial to distinguish biofertilizers from organic fertilizers, which consist of organic compounds that directly enhance soil fertility or do so through decomposition. Not all phosphate solubilizing bacteria (PSB) and plant-growth promoting bacteria meet the criteria for biofertilizers. If their mode of influencing plant growth revolves around controlling harmful organisms, they are categorized as biopesticides instead. To qualify as a biofertilizer, a substance must contain living microorganisms that stimulate plant growth by enriching the plant's nutrient status. A notably higher concentration of PSB, primarily from the genera *Pseudomonas* and *Bacillus*, is commonly observed in the rhizosphere compared to non-rhizospheric soil, as detailed by Misra et al. (2012).

3.5.2 IMPORTANCE

Phosphate solubilizing bacteria (PSB) have gained increasing significance in the agricultural production of specific crops. However, the commercialization and widespread utilization of PSB face limitations, as consistent responses across different host cultivars and various field sites have not been uniformly observed. Additionally, their applications extend to environmental endeavors, such as facilitating re-vegetation in eroded deserts. Despite the promising potential of using PSB in agriculture and addressing environmental challenges, there exists a knowledge gap that hinders their practical implementation. Insufficient understanding of these bacteria necessitates further comprehensive research before establishing their utility in benefiting mankind.

3.5.3 PSB AS BIOCONTROL AGENTS

Phosphate solubilizing bacteria (PSB) as Biocontrol Agents: PSB exhibit the capability to produce substances that confer protection against various diseases. Their function in protecting plants from pathogens entails both direct antagonistic interactions with the pathogen and the stimulation of host resistance. The recent focus on siderophore-producing plant growth-promoting rhizobacteria (PGPR) in the biocontrol of soil-borne plant pathogens has sparked significant interest in microbiological research. Microbiologists have devised methodologies for introducing siderophore-producing PGPR into the soil system through seeds, soil, or root systems. PGPR, which indirectly enhances plant growth by suppressing phytopathogens, employs diverse mechanisms for achieving this effect. These mechanisms include:

- Proficiency in siderophore production, as elucidated previously, wherein the chelation of iron occurs, rendering it inaccessible to pathogens.
- The capability to biosynthesize anti-fungal metabolites, including antibiotics, enzymes that lyse fungal cell walls, or hydrogen cyanide, thereby exerting inhibitory effects on the proliferation of fungal pathogens.
- The aptitude for effective competition with pathogens in the acquisition of nutrients or specific root niches, coupled with the capacity to induce systemic resistance.

Several prominent PSB strains, employed as biofertilizers and biocontrol agents to enhance agricultural productivity, include *Bacillus, Achromobacter, Agrobacterium, Micrococcus, Burkholderia, Erwinia, Flavobacterium, Pseudomonas*, and *Rhizobium* (Srivastava and Shalini, 2009; Tamilarasi et al., 2008). Notably, *Pseudomonas fluorescens* stands out as one of the extensively studied rhizobacteria due to its antagonistic properties against various plant pathogens. In the context of agricultural challenges, Shankar (2013) reported the severe impact of Banana bunchy top virus (BBTV) on banana (*Musa* spp.) crops in the Western Ghats of Tamil Nadu, India. It has been demonstrated that the application of the *P. fluorescens* strain significantly reduced the incidence of BBTV in hill banana, both in greenhouse and field conditions.

3.6 CONCLUSION

The widespread use of chemical phosphorus (P) fertilizers poses a considerable risk to microbial diversity, soil microbial community composition, and soil fertility across various agro-ecosystems, thereby affecting crop yields on a global scale. Given the prevalent deficiency of plant-available P in soils worldwide and the costliness of phosphatic fertilizers, researchers are actively seeking alternatives to address these challenges. Utilizing phosphate solubilizing bacteria (PSB) for plant disease control emerges as a promising avenue for achieving sustainable agriculture goals. To effectively incorporate PSB into sustainable agricultural systems, a comprehensive understanding of their functional diversity, colonizing capabilities, mode of actions, and strategic application is essential. This review delves into various soil microorganisms exhibiting phosphorus solubilization capabilities, positioning them as potential biofertilizers. Emphasis is placed on elucidating the mechanisms involved in inorganic phosphate solubilization by PSB and organic phosphorus mineralization. Additionally, key factors influencing the success of this technology are explored. Ultimately, the adoption of PSB holds promise for promoting sustainable agriculture, and it is asserted that this technology is ripe for commercial exploitation across diverse regions worldwide. The intricate microbial interactions at the soil-root interface (rhizosphere) assume a pivotal role in nutrient transformations, mobilization, and solubilization from the soil nutrient pool, ensuring the uptake of vital nutrients by crop plants. Moreover, these root-associated microorganisms serve as a natural check against the growth and proliferation of various soil-borne pathogens.

KEYWORDS

- **banana bunchy top virus**
- **fertilizers**
- **mineralization**
- **organic phosphorus**
- **phosphate solubilizing bacteria**
- **rhizosphere**
- **solubilization**

REFERENCES

Afzal, A., Ashraf, M., Asad, S. A., & Farooq, M. (2005). Effect of phosphate solubilizing microorganisms on phosphorus uptake, yield and yield traits of wheat (*Triticum aestivum* L.) in rain fed area. *International Journal of Agriculture and Biology*, *7*(2), 207–209.

Ahemad, M. (2014). Phosphate-solubilizing bacteria-assisted phytoremediation of metalliferous soils: A review. Department of Agricultural Microbiology, Faculty of Agricultural Sciences, Aligarh Muslim University, Aligarh 202002, UP, India.

Ahemad, M., & Khan, M. (2011a). Toxicological assessment of selective pesticides towards plant growth promoting activities of phosphate solubilizing *Pseudomonas aeruginosa*. *Acta Microbiological et Immunologica Hungarica*, *58*, 169–187.

Ahemad, M., & Khan, M. S. (2010a). Influence of selective herbicides on plant growth promoting traits of phosphate solubilizing *Enterobacter asburiae* strain PS2. *Research Journal of Microbiology*, *5*, 849–857.

Ahemad, M., & Khan, M. S. (2010b). Plant growth promoting activities of phosphate-solubilizing *Enterobacter asburiae* as influenced by fungicides. *Eurasian Journal of Biosciences*, *4*, 88–95.

Ahemad, M., & Khan, M. S. (2010c). Phosphate-solubilizing and plant growth-promoting *Pseudomonas aeruginosa* PS1 improves greengram performance in quizalafop-p-ethyl and clodinafop amended soil. *Archives of Environmental Contamination and Toxicology*, *58*, 361–372.

Ahemad, M., & Khan, M. S. (2011b). Effects of insecticides on plant growth-promoting activities of phosphate solubilizing rhizobacterium *Klebsiella* sp. strain PS19. *Pesticide Biochemistry and Physiology*, *100*, 51–56.

Ahemad, M., & Khan, M. S. (2011c). Assessment of plant growth promoting activities of rhizobacterium *Pseudomonas putida* under insecticide stress. *Microbiology Journal*, *1*, 54–64.

Ahemad, M., & Khan, M. S. (2011d). Toxicological effects of selective herbicides on plant growth promoting activities of phosphate solubilizing *Klebsiella* sp. strain PS19. *Current Microbiology*, *62*, 532–538.

Ahemad, M., & Khan, M. S. (2011e). *Pseudomonas aeruginosa* strain PS1 enhances growth parameters of green gram [*Vigna radiata* (L.) Wilczek] in insecticide-stressed soils. *Journal of Pest Science, 84*, 123–131.

Ahemad, M., & Khan, M. S. (2012a). Biotoxic impact of fungicides on plant growth promoting activities of phosphate-solubilizing *Klebsiella* sp. isolated from mustard (*Brassica campestris*) rhizosphere. *Journal of Pest Science, 85*, 29–36.

Ahmed, M. F., Kennedy, I. R., Choudhury, A. T. M. A., Kecskes, M. L., & Deker, R. (2008). Phosphorus adsorption in some Australian soils and influence of bacteria on the desorption of phosphorus. *Communications in Soil Science and Plant Analysis, 39*, 1269–1294.

Alam, S., Khalil, S., Ayub, N., & Rashid, M. (2002). *In vitro* solubilization of inorganic phosphate by phosphate solubilizing microorganism (PSM) from maize rhizosphere. *International Journal of Agriculture and Biology, 4*, 454–458.

Babana, A. H., Dicko, A. H., Maïga, K., & Traoré, D. (2013). Characterization of rock phosphate-solubilizing microorganisms isolated from wheat (*Triticum aestivum* L.) rhizosphere in Mali. *Journal of Microbiology and Microbial Research, 1*(1), 1–6.

Bhattacharyya, P., & Jha, D. (2012). Plant growth-promoting rhizobacteria (PGPR): Emergence in agriculture. *World Journal of Microbiology and Biotechnology*, 1–24.

Caron, M., Patten, C. L., & Ghosh, S. (1995). Effects of plant growth promoting rhizobacteria *Pseudomonas putida* GR-122 on the physiology of canola roots. *Plant Growth Regulation Society of America, 22nd Proceedings*, July 18–20, Ed. Green D. W.

Chen, Y. P., Rekha, P. D., Arunshen, A. B., Lai, W. A., & Young, C. C. (2006). Phosphate solubilizing bacteria from subtropical soil and their tricalcium phosphate solubilizing abilities. *Applied Soil Ecology, 34*, 33–41.

Davies, P. J. (1995). *Plant Hormones: Physiology, Biochemistry and Molecular Biology* (2nd ed.). Dordrecht: Kluwer Academic Publishers.

Deubel, A., & Merbach, W. (2005). Influence of microorganisms on phosphorus bioavailability in soils. In Buscot, F., & Varma, A. (Eds.), *Microorganisms in Soils: Roles in Genesis and Functions* (pp. 177–191). Springer-Verlag: Berlin-Heidelberg, Germany.

Duponnois, R., Kisa, M., & Plenchette, C. (2006). Phosphate solubilizing potential of the nematofungus *Arthrobotrys oligospora*. *Journal of Plant Nutrition and Soil Science, 169*, 280–282.

Fankem, H., Nwaga, D., Deubel, A., Dieng, L., Merbach, W., & Etoa, F. X. (2006). Occurrence and functioning of phosphate-solubilizing microorganisms from oil palm tree (*Elaeis guineensis*) rhizosphere in Cameroon. *African Journal of Biotechnology, 5*, 2450–2460.

Gaur, A. C. (1990). *Phosphate Solubilizing Microorganisms as Biofertilizers*. Omega Scientific Publishers: New Delhi. p. 176.

Glick, B. R., Cheng, Z., Czarny, J., & Duan, J. (2007). Promotion of plant growth by ACC deaminase-producing soil bacteria. *European Journal of Plant Pathology, 119*, 329–339.

Gyaneshwar, P., Kumar, G. N., Parekh, L. J., & Poole, P. S. (2002). Role of soil microorganisms in improving P nutrition of plants. *Plant and Soil, 245*, 83–93.

He, L. Y., Zhang, Y. F., Ma, H. Y., Su, L. N., Chen, Z. J., Wang, Q. Y., Meng, Q., & Fang, S. X. (2010). Characterization of copper-resistant bacteria and assessment of bacterial communities in rhizosphere soils of copper-tolerant plants. *Applied Soil Ecology, 44*, 49–55.

Karuppiah, P., & Rajaram, S. (2011). Exploring the potential of chromium-reducing *Bacillus* sp. and their plant growth promoting activities. *Journal of Microbiology Research, 1*, 17–23.

Kucey, R. M. N., Janzen, H. H., & Leggett, M. E. (1989). Microbial mediated increases in plant available phosphorus. *Advances in Agronomy, 42*, 199–228.

Lamo, K., Korla, B. N., & Shukla, Y. R. (2012). Effect of different organic and inorganic sources on seed production of radish (*Raphanus sativus* CV. Chinese pink). *Life Sciences Leaflets, 2*, 38–44.

Li, K., & Ramakrishna, W. (2011). Effect of multiple metal-resistant bacteria from contaminated lake sediments on metal accumulation and plant growth. *Journal of Hazardous Materials, 189*, 531–539.

Mirza, M. S., Ahmad, W., & Latif, F. (2001). Isolation, partial characterization, and the effect of plant growth-promoting bacteria (PGPB) on micro-propagated sugarcane *in vitro*. *Plant and Soil, 237*, 47–54.

Mishra, D. J., Singh, R., Mishra, U. K., & Shahi, S. K. (2012). Role of biofertilizer in organic agriculture: A review. *Journal of Recent Science, 2*(1), 39–41.

Misra, N., Gupta, G., & Jha, P. N. (2012). Assessment of mineral phosphate-solubilizing properties and molecular characterization of zinc-tolerant bacteria. *Journal of Basic Microbiology, 52*, 549–558.

Mohammadi, K. (2011). *Soil, Plant and Microbe Interaction.* Lambert Academic Publishing. 120 pp.

Neal, J. L., Larson, R. I., & Atkinson, T. G. (1973). Changes in rhizosphere populations of selected physiological groups of bacteria related to substitution of specific pairs of chromosomes in spring wheat. *Plant and Soil, 39*, 209–212.

Oves, M., Khan, M. S., & Zaidi, A. (2013). Chromium-reducing and plant growth promoting novel strain *Pseudomonas aeruginosa* OSG41 enhances chickpea growth in chromium-amended soils. *European Journal of Soil Biology, 56*, 72–83.

Ponmurugan, P. C., & Gopi, C. (2006). *In vitro* production of growth regulators and phosphate activity by phosphate-solubilizing bacteria. *African Journal of Biotechnology, 5*, 348–350.

Poonguzhali, S., Madhaiyan, M., & Sa, T. (2008). Isolation and identification of phosphate-solubilizing bacteria from Chinese cabbage and their effect on growth and phosphorus utilization of plants. *Journal of Microbiology and Biotechnology, 18*, 773–777.

Ramkumar, V. S., & Kannapiran, E. (2011). Isolation of total heterotrophic bacteria and phosphate-solubilizing bacteria and *in vitro* study of phosphatase activity and production of phytohormones by PSB. *Archives of Applied Science Research, 3*, 581–586.

Rashid, M. K., Samina, A., Najma, A., Sadia, & Farooq, L. (2004). Organic acids production and phosphate solubilization by phosphate-solubilizing microorganisms under *in vitro* conditions. *Pakistan Journal of Biological Sciences, 7*, 187–196.

Reyes, V. A., & Valduz, Z. (2006). Phosphate-solubilizing microorganisms isolated from the rhizosphere and bulk soils of colonizer plants at an abandoned rock phosphate mine. *Plant and Soil, 287*(12), 69–75.

Salamone, I. E. G., Hynes, R. K., & Nelson, L. M. (2005). Role of cytokinins in plant growth promotion by rhizosphere bacteria. In Siddiqui, Z. A. (Ed.), *PGPR: Biocontrol and Biofertilization* (pp. 173–195). Springer: Amsterdam, The Netherlands.

Sandip, B., Subrata, P., & Swati, R. G. (2011). Isolation and characterization of plant growth-promoting *Bacillus thuringiensis* from agricultural soil of West Bengal. *Research Journal of Biotechnology, 6*, 9–13.

Sharma, R. A., & Parmar, B. B. (1997). Influence of biofertilizers and indigenous sources of nutrients on nutrient uptake and productivity of rainfed soybean–gram cropping sequence. *Crop Research, 13*, 13–18.

Sharma, S. B., Sayyed, R. Z., Trivedi, M. H., & Gobi, T. A. (2013). Phosphate solubilizing microbes: Sustainable approach for managing phosphorus deficiency in agricultural soils. *Springer Plus, 2*, 587–600.

Sharma, S. K., Johri, B. N., Ramesh, A., Joshi, O. P., & Prasad, S. V. S. (2011). Selection of plant growth-promoting *Pseudomonas* spp. that enhanced productivity of soybean–wheat cropping system in central India. *Journal of Microbiology and Biotechnology, 21*, 1127–1142.

Sharpley, A. (2006). Agricultural phosphorus management: Protecting production and water quality. *Agricultural Phosphate Management: Protecting Production and Water Quality, Lesson 34*. USDA-Agricultural Research Service, MidWest Plant Service. Iowa State University, Ames. http://www.lpes.org/Lessons/Lessons34/34-PhosphorusManagement.html (accessed on 2nd January 2026).

Shrivastava, R., & Shalini. (2009). Antifungal activity of *Pseudomonas fluorescens* against pathogenic fungi. *The Internet Journal of Microbiology*, *7*(2).

Singh, J. S. (2013). Plant growth promoting rhizobacteria: Potential microbes for sustainable agriculture. *Article*, 275–281.

Sobral, J. K. (2003). *A Comunidade Bacteriana Endofítica Epifítica De Soja (Glycine max) e Estudo da Interação Endófitos-Planta* [Dissertation, São Paulo State University].

Swaby, R., & Sperber, J. I. (1958). Phosphate dissolving microorganisms in the rhizosphere of legume. In *Nutrition of Legumes: Proceedings of the 5th Easter School in Agricultural Science, University of Nottingham* (pp. 289–294). CSIRO Adelaide. *Soils and Fertilizers* (1959).

Tamilarasi, S., Lakshmanaperumalsamy, P., Nanthakumar, K., & Karthikeyan, K. (2006). Diversity of root-associated microorganisms of selected medicinal plants and influence of rhizo-microorganisms on the antimicrobial property of *Coriandrum sativum*. *Journal of Environmental Biology, 29*(1), 127–134.

Upadhayay, A., & Srivastava, S. (2012). Evaluation of multiple plant growth-promoting traits of an isolate of *Pseudomonas fluorescens* strain Psd. *Indian Journal of Experimental Biology, 48*, 601–609.

van Peer, R., Niemann, G. J., & Schippers, B. (1991). Induced resistance and phytoalexin accumulation in biological control of *Fusarium* wilt of carnation by *Pseudomonas* sp. strain WCS417r. *Phytopathology, 81*, 728–734.

Vessey, J. K. (2003). Plant growth promoting rhizobacteria as biofertilizers. *Plant and Soil, 255*, 571–586.

Vlek, P. L. G., & Vielhauer, K. (1994). Nutrient management strategies in stressed environments. In Virmani, S. M., Katyal, J. C., Eswaran, H., & Abrol, I. P. (Eds.), *Stressed Ecosystems and Sustainable Agriculture* (pp. 203–229). Oxford and IBH Publishing Co., New Delhi, India.

Wani, P. A., & Khan, M. S. (2010). *Bacillus* species enhance growth parameters of chickpea (*Cicer arietinum* L.) in chromium-stressed soils. *Food and Chemical Toxicology, 48*, 3262–3267.

Whitelaw, M. A. (2000). Growth promotion of plants inoculated with phosphate-solubilizing fungi. *Advances in Agronomy, 69*, 99–151.

Yasmin, H., & Bano, A. (2011). Isolation and characterization of phosphate-solubilizing bacteria from rhizosphere soil of Khewra Salt Range and Attock. *Pakistan Journal of Botany, 43*, 1663–1668.

CHAPTER 4

Liquid Biofertilizers for Sustainable Agriculture: Formulations and Technologies

PRITI PAL,[1] PRAKASH KUMAR SARANGI,[2] OM PRAKASH,[3] ANAND PRAKASH,[3] UTTAM KUMAR SAHOO,[4] BRIJESH PANDEY,[3] and AKHILESH KUMAR SINGH[3,*]

[1]*Amity Institute of Biotechnology, Amity University Uttar Pradesh, Lucknow Campus, Lucknow, India*

[2]*College of Agriculture, Central Agricultural University, Imphal, Manipur, India*

[3]*Department of Biotechnology, School of Life Sciences, Mahatma Gandhi Central University, Motihari, Bihar, India*

[4]*Department of Forestry, Mizoram University, Aizawl, Mizoram, India*

*Corresponding authors

ABSTRACT

In the pursuit of sustainable agricultural practices, liquid biofertilizers have emerged as a promising and eco-friendly alternative to traditional chemical fertilizers. This abstract provides a concise overview of the key aspects surrounding liquid biofertilizers, focusing on their composition, mechanisms of action, and implications for sustainable agriculture. Liquid biofertilizers consist of microbial agents such as nitrogen-fixing bacteria, phosphorus-solubilizing bacteria, and potassium-mobilizing bacteria, which play pivotal roles in enhancing soil fertility and nutrient availability. The chapter explores the intricate mechanisms through

Biotechnology for Sustainable Agriculture: Innovative Approaches and Strategies.
Prakash Kumar Sarangi (Ed)

DOI: 10.1201/9781779642998-4

which these microorganisms contribute to nitrogen fixation, phosphorus solubilization, and potassium mobilization, promoting optimal plant growth and development. Despite their potential, challenges such as shelf life and compatibility with other inputs are addressed, emphasizing the need for further research and technological innovations to optimize their effectiveness. Drawing from case studies, the abstract highlights successful implementations and acknowledges existing challenges. Looking forward, the abstract suggests future prospects, including emerging technologies and research directions, reinforcing the pivotal role of liquid biofertilizers in fostering sustainable agriculture practices for a resilient and environmentally conscious future.

4.1 INTRODUCTION

As humanity navigates the complex terrain of the 21st century, the agricultural sector finds itself at the crossroads of unprecedented challenges and opportunities. The quest for sustainable agricultural practices has become imperative, driven by the need to feed a burgeoning global population while mitigating the environmental impacts of conventional farming methods. In this context, the exploration and utilization of innovative solutions, such as liquid biofertilizers, have garnered significant attention for their potential to revolutionize the agricultural landscape (Allouzi et al., 2022). Traditional agriculture, marked by the widespread use of chemical fertilizers and pesticides, has undoubtedly played a crucial role in meeting the growing demands for food. However, this success has come at a considerable cost. Excessive reliance on chemical inputs has led to soil degradation, water pollution, and a decline in biodiversity. The detrimental effects of these practices have become increasingly evident, prompting a paradigm shift towards sustainable agriculture (Cha et al., 2021).

Sustainable agriculture, in essence, seeks to balance the need for increased food production with environmental stewardship and social responsibility. It encompasses a holistic approach that considers the long-term health of ecosystems, the well-being of farmers, and the resilience of agricultural systems in the face of climate change. Within this framework, the role of fertilizers is pivotal, as they directly influence soil fertility, crop productivity, and environmental sustainability (Wable and Khandelwal, 2023). Liquid biofertilizers represent a departure from the conventional, synthetic inputs that have dominated agricultural practices for decades. Comprising living microorganisms, these biofertilizers introduce a dynamic and symbiotic element to the soil-plant system. Nitrogen-fixing bacteria, phosphorus-solubilizing bacteria, and potassium-mobilizing bacteria, among other beneficial microbes, form the core constituents of these liquid formulations (Kumar et al., 2022).

The appeal of liquid biofertilizers lies in their ability to harness the power of nature's own nutrient cycling processes. Unlike chemical fertilizers that deliver nutrients in a readily available form, liquid biofertilizers rely on microbial activity to convert atmospheric nitrogen into plant-usable forms, solubilize phosphorus bound in the soil, and mobilize potassium for enhanced plant uptake. This biological approach aligns with the principles of sustainable agriculture, fostering a more harmonious relationship between agriculture and the environment (Varshini and Jayanthi, 2020).

4.2 COMPONENTS OF LIQUID BIOFERTILIZERS: MICROBIAL ALCHEMISTS IN AGRICULTURE

To understand the transformative potential of liquid biofertilizers, it is essential to delve into the microscopic realm of nitrogen-fixing bacteria, phosphorus-solubilizing bacteria, and potassium-mobilizing bacteria. These microbial agents act as alchemists in the soil, catalyzing processes that unlock essential nutrients for plant growth. Nitrogen-fixing bacteria, commonly of the genera Rhizobium and Azotobacter, have the remarkable ability to convert atmospheric nitrogen into ammonia—a form that plants can readily assimilate (Meena et al., 2021). This symbiotic relationship between nitrogen-fixing bacteria and leguminous plants exemplifies the elegance of nature's nitrogen cycle, reducing the need for synthetic nitrogen fertilizers. Phosphorus-solubilizing bacteria, such as those from the genera Bacillus and Pseudomonas, play a critical role in enhancing phosphorus availability in the soil (Arfarita et al., 2020). By secreting organic acids and enzymes, these bacteria break down insoluble phosphates, making phosphorus more accessible to plant roots. This mechanism not only improves nutrient uptake but also addresses the issue of phosphorus immobilization in many soils. Potassium-mobilizing bacteria, including species like *Bacillus mucilaginosus*, assist in releasing bound potassium, promoting its movement in the soil and increasing its availability to plants (Kumawat et al., 2021). Potassium is an essential nutrient for various physiological processes in plants, including water uptake, enzyme activation, and disease resistance. The role of these bacteria in mobilizing potassium contributes to overall plant health and resilience. In addition to these primary microbial agents, liquid biofertilizers may also contain a diverse array of other beneficial microorganisms, including mycorrhizal fungi and plant growth-promoting rhizobacteria (PGPR). These microorganisms establish symbiotic relationships with plants, enhancing nutrient absorption, root development, and stress tolerance (Krishnaprabu, 2020).

4.3 MECHANISMS OF ACTION: MICROBIAL CHOREOGRAPHY IN NUTRIENT DYNAMICS

The effectiveness of liquid biofertilizers lies in the intricate dance of microbial communities within the soil. Understanding the mechanisms through which these microorganisms operate provides insights into the dynamic processes that contribute to sustainable nutrient management (Asha et al., 2023).

4.3.1 NITROGEN FIXATION: UNLOCKING ATMOSPHERIC NITROGEN

Nitrogen, a fundamental element for plant growth, is abundant in the atmosphere but largely inaccessible to plants in its gaseous form (Figure 4.1). Nitrogen-fixing bacteria, through a fascinating symbiosis with leguminous plants or free-living in the soil, convert atmospheric nitrogen into ammonia. This ammonia is then further transformed into ammonium ions, a form readily taken up by plant roots. The process not only provides plants with a vital nutrient but also reduces the need for synthetic nitrogen fertilizers, mitigating the environmental impact associated with their production and use (Yadav and Sarkar, 2019).

4.3.2 PHOSPHORUS SOLUBILIZATION: LIBERATING BOUND PHOSPHATES

Phosphorus, crucial for energy transfer in plants, is often present in the soil in insoluble forms. Phosphorus-solubilizing bacteria employ a suite of biochemical mechanisms to break down these insoluble phosphates, releasing soluble forms of phosphorus into the soil solution. This enhances the availability of

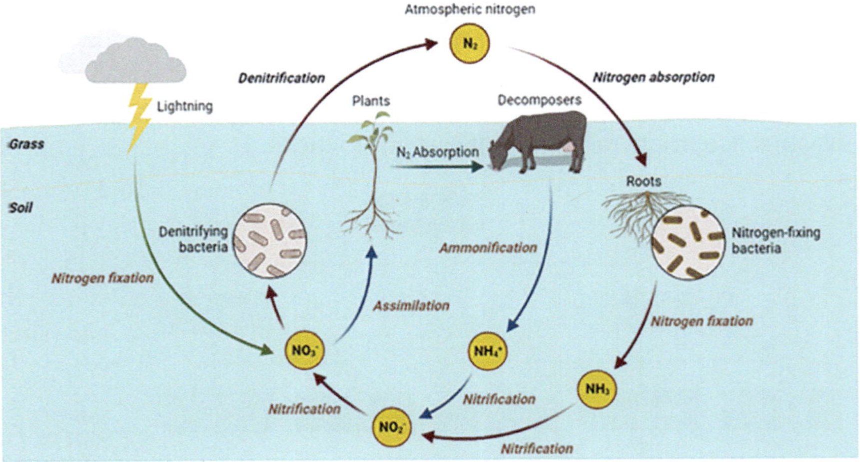

FIGURE 4.1 Nitrogen fixation: Tapping into atmospheric nitrogen reservoirs.

phosphorus for plant uptake, promoting root development, flowering, and fruiting (Patel and Goswami, 2020). By facilitating the solubilization of bound phosphates, these bacteria contribute to sustainable phosphorus management and alleviate the need for excessive phosphorus fertilization.

4.3.3 POTASSIUM MOBILIZATION: ENHANCING PLANT UPTAKE

Potassium, essential for osmoregulation, enzyme activation, and overall plant health, is often tightly bound in the soil. Potassium-mobilizing bacteria produce organic acids that dissolve soil minerals, releasing potassium ions into the soil solution. This mobilization makes potassium more accessible to plant roots, supporting critical physiological processes. The increased availability of potassium contributes to enhanced water uptake, disease resistance, and improved overall plant vigor.

4.3.4 SYNERGISTIC EFFECTS: THE POWER OF MICROBIAL COMMUNITIES

While each microbial agent plays a distinct role, the true power of liquid biofertilizers lies in the synergistic effects of these microorganisms working together. Nitrogen-fixing bacteria, phosphorus-solubilizing bacteria, and potassium-mobilizing bacteria interact in a complex web of relationships, with each microbial community influencing the other. This microbial choreography results in a holistic improvement in soil health, nutrient availability, and plant resilience (Etesami et al., 2017). The intricate interplay between these microorganisms contributes to a balanced and sustainable nutrient management system (Figure 4.2).

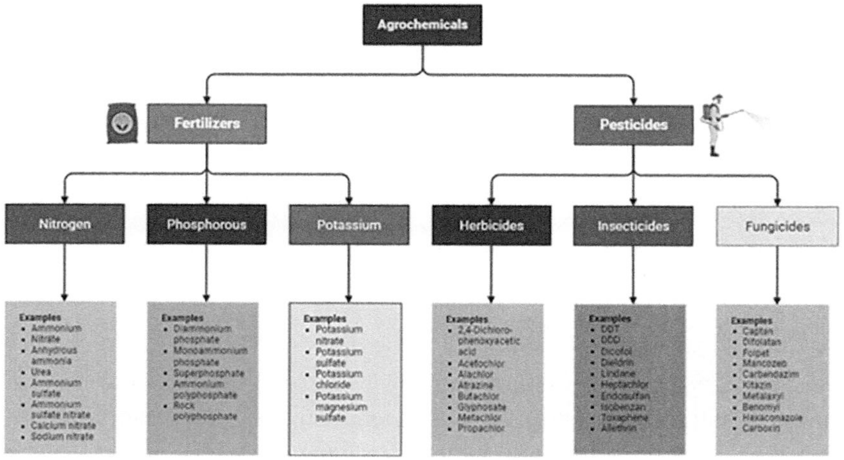

FIGURE 4.2 Application of pesticides by farmers cultivating crops.

4.4 ADVANTAGES OF LIQUID BIOFERTILIZERS: CULTIVATING SUSTAINABLE AGRICULTURE

In the endeavor to redefine agriculture through a lens of sustainability, liquid biofertilizers emerge as a beacon of promise, offering a multitude of advantages that extend far beyond the conventional boundaries of productivity (Allouzi et al., 2022). This section delves into the comprehensive array of benefits that liquid biofertilizers bring to the forefront of modern agricultural practices, encompassing environmental, economic, and agronomic dimensions.

4.4.1 ENVIRONMENTAL BENEFITS

1. **Reduced Chemical Dependency:** One of the primary environmental advantages of liquid biofertilizers lies in their capacity to reduce the dependency on chemical fertilizers. Traditional fertilizers, rich in synthetic nutrients, often contribute to soil degradation and water pollution. Liquid biofertilizers, with their reliance

on beneficial microorganisms, promote a more balanced nutrient supply, minimizing the environmental footprint associated with chemical inputs (Pogula, 2018).

2. **Mitigation of Soil and Water Pollution:** The microbial-driven nutrient release in liquid biofertilizers reduces the risk of nutrient leaching and runoff, addressing a significant concern in conventional agriculture. Nitrogen-fixing bacteria, for instance, facilitate the conversion of atmospheric nitrogen into plant-available forms, reducing the need for nitrogen-based synthetic fertilizers (Pogula, 2018). This, in turn, mitigates the potential for nitrogen runoff, a major contributor to water pollution. By adopting liquid biofertilizers, farmers contribute to the preservation of water quality and the health of aquatic ecosystems (Peta, 2020).
3. **Enhanced Soil Structure and Fertility:** Liquid biofertilizers play a pivotal role in enhancing soil structure and fertility. The activities of phosphorus-solubilizing bacteria contribute to the breakdown of insoluble phosphates, releasing phosphorus into the soil. This not only improves nutrient availability but also enhances soil structure, fostering better water retention and aeration (Mukherjee et al., 2023). The overall improvement in soil health creates a conducive environment for plant growth while reducing the need for soil amendments.
4. **Microbial Diversity and Ecosystem Balance:** The application of liquid biofertilizers introduces a diverse consortium of beneficial microorganisms into the soil ecosystem. This microbial diversity contributes to the overall balance of the soil microbiome, preventing the dominance of harmful pathogens and promoting a symbiotic relationship between plants and microbes (Singh and Vyas, 2016). As a result, the ecosystem becomes more resilient to diseases and pests, reducing the necessity for chemical interventions and fostering a healthier and more sustainable agricultural environment.

4.4.2 ECONOMIC BENEFITS

1. **Cost-Effectiveness:** Liquid biofertilizers offer economic advantages to farmers, primarily through cost-effectiveness. While the initial investment in these biofertilizers may require

some consideration, the long-term benefits often outweigh the costs. Reduced reliance on expensive chemical fertilizers, coupled with increased crop yields and quality, translates into economic gains for farmers (Ammar et al., 2023). This cost-effectiveness is particularly significant for small-scale farmers with limited financial resources.

2. **Improved Crop Yields and Quality:** The application of liquid biofertilizers has been correlated with improved crop yields and enhanced produce quality. The symbiotic relationships established between plants and nitrogen-fixing bacteria, phosphorus-solubilizing bacteria, and potassium-mobilizing bacteria contribute to optimal nutrient availability (Çakmakçı, 2019). This, in turn, results in robust plant growth, increased flowering, and improved fruiting. The overall improvement in crop health and yield directly impacts the economic viability of farming operations.

3. **Reduced Input Costs:** Liquid biofertilizers play a role in reducing the overall input costs associated with agriculture. The microbial processes involved in nutrient release contribute to a more sustainable nutrient cycling system, reducing the need for frequent and high doses of chemical fertilizers (Yadav, 2018). Additionally, the improved soil structure and microbial diversity may decrease the reliance on pesticides and other agrochemicals, further lowering input costs and contributing to the economic efficiency of farming practices.

4. **Market Access and Premium Pricing:** As consumer awareness of sustainable and eco-friendly agricultural practices grows, there is an increasing demand for produce cultivated using environmentally conscious methods. Farmers employing liquid biofertilizers may find themselves in a favorable position in the market, attracting consumers who prioritize sustainably produced food (Handayani et al., 2021). This, in turn, opens avenues for market access and potentially premium pricing for crops grown with biofertilizers, offering an economic incentive for farmers to adopt these sustainable practices.

4.4.3 AGRONOMIC BENEFITS

1. **Enhanced Nutrient Uptake:** The fundamental role of liquid biofertilizers lies in their ability to enhance nutrient uptake by plants. Nitrogen-fixing bacteria, by converting atmospheric nitrogen into plant-usable forms, provide a sustainable source of nitrogen. Phosphorus-solubilizing bacteria make phosphorus more accessible to plant roots, and potassium-mobilizing bacteria enhance the availability of potassium. This synergistic action results in improved nutrient absorption by plants, fostering their overall health and vitality (Ahirwar et al., 2020).

2. **Stimulated Root Development:** The microbial interactions facilitated by liquid biofertilizers contribute to enhanced root development in plants. The secretion of growth-promoting substances by certain bacteria and fungi in these formulations stimulates root elongation and branching. A well-developed root system improves nutrient and water absorption, making plants more resilient to environmental stresses such as drought (Kumawat et al., 2021). This agronomic benefit is crucial for sustainable agriculture, especially in regions prone to water scarcity.

3. **Disease Suppression:** The introduction of beneficial microorganisms into the soil through liquid biofertilizers plays a role in suppressing soil-borne diseases. Antagonistic interactions between beneficial microorganisms and pathogenic species help create a microbial balance that inhibits the proliferation of harmful pathogens. This natural disease suppression reduces the need for chemical pesticides, aligning with the principles of integrated pest management (IPM) and contributing to the sustainability of agricultural ecosystems (Tyagi et al., 2019).

4. **Adaptability to Various Crops:** Liquid biofertilizers exhibit versatility in their application across a wide range of crops. From cereals and pulses to fruits and vegetables, these biofertilizers can be adapted to suit the specific nutrient requirements of different crops (Upadhaya et al., 2022). This adaptability is crucial for promoting sustainable agricultural practices on a large scale, offering a holistic solution that transcends the limitations of single-crop-focused fertilization strategies.

4.4.4 SOCIAL BENEFITS

1. **Healthier Food Production:** The adoption of liquid biofertilizers contributes to the production of healthier and more nutrient-dense food. The balanced nutrient supply facilitated by these biofertilizers enhances the nutritional content of crops, providing consumers with food that is not only abundant but also nutritionally rich (Das et al., 2019). This is particularly significant in addressing global concerns related to malnutrition and food security.
2. **Improved Livelihoods for Farmers:** The economic benefits derived from the adoption of liquid biofertilizers translate into improved livelihoods for farmers. By reducing input costs, improving crop yields, and potentially accessing premium markets, farmers practicing sustainable agriculture with biofertilizers can achieve better economic stability (Jin et al., 2020). This, in turn, has positive implications for rural communities, contributing to poverty alleviation and improved quality of life.
3. **Empowering Small-Scale Farmers:** The cost-effectiveness and adaptability of liquid biofertilizers make them particularly empowering for small-scale farmers. These farmers, often operating with limited resources, can benefit from sustainable agricultural practices that optimize input efficiency and reduce environmental impact (Gul et al., 2019). The social dimension of liquid biofertilizer adoption extends to empowering smallholders to participate more actively in sustainable agriculture.

4.5 APPLICATION TECHNIQUES OF LIQUID BIOFERTILIZERS FOR SUSTAINABLE AGRICULTURE

The efficacy of liquid biofertilizers in promoting sustainable agriculture is not solely dependent on their composition but is intricately tied to the methods of application. Choosing the right application technique ensures optimal interaction between beneficial microorganisms and the plant-soil system (Gulshan et al., 2022). This section explores various application techniques, emphasizing seed treatment, soil application, and foliar spray, to unravel the versatility and adaptability of liquid biofertilizers in diverse agricultural contexts.

4.5.1 *SEED TREATMENT: NURTURING FROM THE START*

1. **Introduction to Seed Treatment:** Seed treatment with liquid biofertilizers involves coating seeds with a microbial solution before planting. This technique harnesses the symbiotic relationship between seeds and microorganisms, jumpstarting the plant-microbe association from the very beginning of the crop cycle (Gautam et al., 2021). The process is especially effective for crops with seeds that interact closely with soil microorganisms during germination and early growth.

   i. **Benefits of Seed Treatment:**

      a. **Early Root Colonization:** Coating seeds with liquid biofertilizers facilitates early colonization of the developing root system by beneficial microorganisms. This preemptive establishment of a microbial community around the roots enhances nutrient availability and primes the plant for a symbiotic relationship throughout its life cycle (Singh et al., 2020).

      b. **Protection Against Pathogens:** The introduction of beneficial microorganisms through seed treatment can confer protection against soil-borne pathogens. Some microorganisms in biofertilizers produce antimicrobial substances that inhibit the growth of harmful pathogens, creating a protective zone around the germinating seed and young seedlings (Przygocka-Cyna et al., 2021).

      c. **Improved Germination Rates:** Seed treatment has been linked to improved germination rates. The presence of certain microorganisms stimulates seed germination and early root development, providing a competitive advantage to the emerging seedlings (Dilnashin et al., 2020).

   ii. **Application Guidelines:**

      a. **Preparation of Seed Coating:** Liquid biofertilizers are typically diluted with water to create a solution suitable for seed coating. The concentration depends on the specific biofertilizer formulation and the targeted crop. Some formulations may also include adhesives or sticking agents to enhance the adherence of the microbial solution to the seed surface (Youssef and Farag, 2021).

b. **Drying Time:** After coating, seeds are left to dry before planting. The drying time allows the microbial solution to adhere firmly to the seed surface, ensuring that the beneficial microorganisms are in close proximity to the emerging roots upon germination.

iii. **Crop-Specific Considerations:**

a. **Leguminous Crops:** Nitrogen-fixing bacteria are often included in seed treatment formulations for leguminous crops. This symbiotic association between nitrogen-fixing bacteria and legume roots is crucial for atmospheric nitrogen fixation, providing a natural source of nitrogen for the leguminous plants (Sahu et al., 2022).

4.5.2 SOIL APPLICATION: NOURISHING THE ROOT ZONE

1. **Introduction to Soil Application:** The application of liquid biofertilizers directly to the soil is a common and versatile technique. This method is suitable for a wide range of crops and is particularly effective for enhancing soil fertility and promoting the overall health of the soil-plant ecosystem (Singh et al., 2019).

i. **Benefits of Soil Application:**

a. **Even Nutrient Distribution:** Soil application ensures even distribution of beneficial microorganisms throughout the root zone. This uniform distribution is vital for establishing a balanced and symbiotic microbial community, contributing to consistent nutrient availability for plant roots.

b. **Long-Term Soil Health:** Regular soil applications of liquid biofertilizers contribute to long-term improvements in soil health. The microbial activity helps in breaking down organic matter, releasing nutrients, and improving soil structure. This, in turn, enhances water retention, aeration, and nutrient-holding capacity.

ii. **Application Guidelines:**

a. **Dilution and Concentration:** Liquid biofertilizers are typically diluted with water before soil application. The concentration of the solution depends on factors such as the crop type, soil conditions, and the specific formulation of the biofertilizer. Recommendations from the biofertilizer manufacturer or agricultural extension services guide the appropriate dilution rates (Panda et al., 2022).

b. **Timing of Application:** The timing of soil application is critical and varies depending on the crop's growth stage. While some liquid biofertilizers can be applied during the early stages of crop development, others are more effective when applied during specific growth phases, such as flowering or fruiting. Understanding the nutrient requirements of the crop and aligning the application with its growth stages is essential for maximizing benefits (Mohanty et al., 2021).

iii. **Crop-Specific Considerations:**

a. **Cereals and Grains:** Soil application is widely employed for cereals and grains, ensuring a steady supply of nutrients during critical growth stages. The phosphorus-solubilizing and potassium-mobilizing capabilities of certain bacteria in biofertilizers are particularly beneficial for these crops.

b. **Fruit Trees and Perennials:** For perennial crops like fruit trees, regular soil application of liquid biofertilizers contributes to sustained nutrient availability. The slow-release nature of nutrients through microbial activity aligns well with the longer life cycle of perennial plants.

4.5.3 FOLIAR SPRAY: DIRECT NUTRIENT ABSORPTION

1. **Introduction to Foliar Spray:** Foliar spray involves the direct application of liquid biofertilizers onto the leaves of plants. This technique is particularly effective for crops with a well-developed leaf surface and is advantageous in situations where rapid nutrient absorption is crucial.

i. Benefits of Foliar Spray:

a. **Quick Nutrient Uptake:** Foliar spray allows for the rapid absorption of nutrients directly through the leaves, providing an immediate boost to plant nutrient levels. This is especially advantageous during critical growth stages when nutrient demand is high.

b. **Addressing Micronutrient Deficiencies:** Foliar application is an effective method for addressing micronutrient deficiencies. Some liquid biofertilizers contain microorganisms that facilitate the solubilization of micronutrients, making them more available for foliar absorption.

c. **Reduced Soil Interference:** By bypassing the soil, foliar spray reduces the interference of soil-related factors that may affect nutrient uptake. This is particularly beneficial in situations where soil conditions are suboptimal or where plants exhibit symptoms of nutrient deficiencies.

ii. Application Guidelines:

a. **Dilution Ratios:** Liquid biofertilizers for foliar spray are generally diluted with water to achieve an optimal concentration. The dilution ratio depends on the specific formulation of the biofertilizer and the targeted crop. Adjuvants such as surfactants may be added to enhance the coverage and adherence of the solution to the leaf surface (Satpute et al., 2021).

b. **Timing and Frequency:** Foliar spray is often applied during specific growth stages, such as vegetative growth, flowering, or fruiting. The frequency of application depends on the nutrient requirements of the crop and environmental conditions. Foliar spray is typically conducted early in the morning or late in the afternoon to avoid adverse weather conditions.

iii. Crop-Specific Considerations:

a. **Horticultural Crops:** Foliar spray is widely utilized in horticultural crops such as vegetables and fruits, where rapid nutrient uptake is crucial for high-quality produce. It is particularly effective for addressing micronutrient deficiencies that can impact fruit quality.

b. **Stressed or Deficient Crops:** Foliar application is beneficial for crops experiencing stress conditions or exhibiting symptoms of nutrient deficiencies. The direct application of nutrients to the leaves provides a quick remedy, bypassing any limitations in the soil.

4.5.4 CHALLENGES AND LIMITATIONS OF LIQUID BIOFERTILIZERS IN SUSTAINABLE AGRICULTURE

While liquid biofertilizers hold immense promise for sustainable agriculture, their widespread adoption is not without challenges and limitations. Understanding these constraints is crucial for developing strategies to optimize the efficacy of biofertilizers and address potential barriers to their integration into mainstream agricultural practices. This section explores the multifaceted challenges associated with liquid biofertilizers, spanning issues related to shelf life, compatibility with other inputs, and the awareness and adoption dynamics among farmers.

1. **Shelf Life and Storage Challenges: Microbial Viability Matters:**

i. **Microbial Viability:** The heart of liquid biofertilizers lies in the microbial agents they contain—nitrogen-fixing bacteria, phosphorus-solubilizing bacteria, and potassium-mobilizing bacteria, among others. Maintaining the viability and activity of these microorganisms is crucial for the effectiveness of the biofertilizer. However, the shelf life of many liquid formulations can be limited, and the survival of microbes can be influenced by various factors.

ii. **Sensitivity to Environmental Conditions:** Microorganisms in liquid biofertilizers can be sensitive to environmental conditions such as temperature, humidity, and exposure to sunlight. Variability in storage conditions, especially during transportation and storage at retail outlets, can impact microbial viability. High temperatures can lead to the deterioration of microbial cells, rendering them less effective upon application.

iii. **Inhibition by Chemicals:** Some chemical components in liquid biofertilizers, such as preservatives or stabilizers, may inadvertently inhibit the activity of beneficial microorganisms. Striking a balance between ensuring the longevity of the product on the shelf and preserving microbial viability is a delicate challenge that biofertilizer manufacturers must address.

iv. **Mitigation Strategies:** Manufacturers are continually working on developing formulations and storage methods that enhance the shelf life of liquid biofertilizers. Encapsulation technologies, protective carriers, and novel packaging methods are being explored to safeguard microbial viability during storage and transportation.

2. **Compatibility with Other Inputs: Navigating Interactions:**

i. **Interaction with Pesticides:** The co-application of liquid biofertilizers with chemical pesticides poses challenges due to potential interactions between the microorganisms and pesticide formulations. Some pesticides may have adverse effects on the viability of beneficial microorganisms, leading to a reduction in their efficacy.

ii. **Competing with Chemical Fertilizers:** Liquid biofertilizers must coexist with chemical fertilizers, as farmers often continue using conventional nutrient inputs. However, the simultaneous application of chemical fertilizers may affect the nutrient release patterns of biofertilizers. Striking a balance to optimize the synergistic effects while avoiding antagonistic interactions is a complex task.

iii. **Adjusting Application Practices:** To address compatibility issues, farmers may need to adjust their application practices, including the timing and method of applying chemical inputs and biofertilizers. Integrated crop management strategies that consider the potential interactions between different inputs are essential for optimizing nutrient availability and crop performance.

iv. **Research and Guidelines:** Research on the compatibility of specific liquid biofertilizer formulations with commonly used pesticides and fertilizers is essential. Clear guidelines and recommendations for farmers regarding the timing and sequence of application can help minimize negative interactions and promote the harmonious coexistence of different agricultural inputs.

3. **Awareness and Adoption Challenges: Breaking Barriers to Acceptance:**

   i. **Lack of Awareness:** Despite the potential benefits, a significant challenge for the widespread adoption of liquid biofertilizers is the lack of awareness among farmers. Many farmers may not be familiar with the concept of biofertilizers, their mechanisms of action, or their potential contributions to sustainable agriculture.

   ii. **Education and Extension Services:** Bridging the awareness gap requires targeted education and extension services. Agricultural extension officers, NGOs, and other stakeholders play a crucial role in disseminating information about the benefits of liquid biofertilizers, providing training on their application, and addressing misconceptions or concerns among farmers.

   iii. **Perceptions and Skepticism:** Farmers may be hesitant to adopt liquid biofertilizers due to skepticism about their effectiveness compared to traditional chemical fertilizers. Perceptions that biofertilizers are less potent or reliable can hinder their adoption, emphasizing the need for robust scientific evidence and successful case studies.

   iv. **Demonstration Farms and Field Trials:** Establishing demonstration farms and conducting field trials can serve as effective tools for showcasing the benefits of liquid biofertilizers in real-world agricultural settings. Farmers are more likely to adopt new practices when they witness tangible improvements in crop performance and yield.

4. **Precision and Application Technology: Fine-Tuning Delivery:**

   i. **Need for Precision Agriculture:** The effective application of liquid biofertilizers requires precision agriculture practices. Precision in dosage, timing, and application methods is essential to maximize the impact of these biofertilizers. However, not all farmers have access to the technology and equipment needed for precision agriculture.

ii. **Investment in Application Technology:** The adoption of precision agriculture technologies, including specialized equipment for the application of liquid biofertilizers, may require significant investment. Small-scale farmers, in particular, may face financial constraints in acquiring and maintaining such technology, limiting their ability to optimize the application process.

iii. **Education on Application Techniques:** Providing farmers with education on optimal application techniques, even without high-tech equipment, is crucial. Simple and practical guidelines for dilution rates, application intervals, and compatibility with existing farm machinery can empower farmers to make the most of liquid biofertilizers.

5. **Quality Control and Standardization: Ensuring Consistency:**

i. **Batch-to-Batch Variability:** The consistency of liquid biofertilizers from batch to batch can be a challenge. Variability in microbial content, nutrient concentrations, and overall formulation can impact the reliability and predictability of results for farmers.

ii. **Quality Control Measures:** Implementing stringent quality control measures in the production and formulation of liquid biofertilizers is essential. Standardizing production processes, monitoring microbial content, and conducting regular quality checks can help minimize batch-to-batch variability.

iii. **Certification and Standards:** Establishing certification standards for liquid biofertilizers can provide assurance to farmers regarding product quality and effectiveness. Industry-wide adherence to standardized practices ensures that farmers receive reliable and consistent products, building trust in the efficacy of biofertilizers.

6. **Regulatory Framework: Navigating Approval Processes:**

i. **Lack of Regulatory Clarity:** In some regions, there may be a lack of clear regulatory frameworks for the registration and approval of liquid biofertilizers. The absence of standardized regulations can create uncertainty for manufacturers, hindering the development and commercialization of new biofertilizer formulations.

ii. **Navigating Approval Processes:** Biofertilizer manufacturers may face challenges in navigating regulatory approval processes, which can be time-consuming and resource-intensive. Developing a streamlined and transparent regulatory framework for biofertilizers can encourage innovation and facilitate their entry into the market.

iii. **Global Harmonization**: Achieving global harmonization in regulatory standards for biofertilizers would promote consistency and facilitate the international trade of these products. Collaborative efforts among regulatory authorities, industry stakeholders, and scientific communities are crucial for establishing coherent and science-based regulations.

4.5.5 FUTURE PROSPECTS AND RESEARCH DIRECTIONS IN LIQUID BIOFERTILIZERS FOR SUSTAINABLE AGRICULTURE

The field of liquid biofertilizers is dynamic and holds considerable promise for the future of sustainable agriculture. As research continues to unravel the intricate interactions between beneficial microorganisms, plants, and soils, and as technology advances, several future prospects and research directions emerge. This section explores key areas of potential growth and innovation in the realm of liquid biofertilizers.

1. **Microbial Technology Advancements: Unlocking the Microbial Black Box:**

i. **Genetic Engineering of Microorganisms:** Advances in genetic engineering techniques offer the potential to enhance the traits of beneficial microorganisms in liquid biofertilizers. Genetic modifications can be designed to optimize nitrogen-fixing capabilities, phosphorus-solubilizing efficiency, and other essential functions, leading to biofertilizers with improved efficacy and specificity for different crops and soil conditions (Mukherjee et al., 2023).

ii. **Synthetic Biology Approaches:** Synthetic biology, with its ability to design and construct biological systems, provides a platform for creating custom-tailored microbial consortia. This approach allows scientists to engineer synthetic communities that work synergistically to enhance nutrient availability, promote plant health, and mitigate environmental stress factors. The application of synthetic biology principles to liquid biofertilizers opens new frontiers for precision agriculture.

iii. **Omics Technologies:** The integration of omics technologies, including genomics, transcriptomics, proteomics, and metabolomics, allows researchers to delve into the molecular mechanisms underlying microbial-plant interactions. Comprehensive profiling of microbial communities and their responses to environmental stimuli provides valuable insights for optimizing biofertilizer formulations and understanding the dynamic nature of soil-plant-microbe interactions.

2. **Nanotechnology Applications: Precision Nutrient Delivery:**

i. **Nanoencapsulation of Microorganisms:** Nanotechnology offers opportunities for the nanoencapsulation of microbial agents in liquid biofertilizers. Nanoencapsulation protects microorganisms from environmental stresses, improves their stability, and enables controlled release of nutrients. This technology has the potential to enhance the shelf life and delivery efficiency of liquid biofertilizers (Jha et al., 2023).

ii. **Nanostructured Nutrient Carriers:** Nanostructured materials can be designed to serve as carriers for nutrients, protecting them from leaching and providing a controlled release in the soil. This approach ensures targeted nutrient delivery to plant roots, minimizing nutrient losses and optimizing nutrient use efficiency (Tallou et al., 2021).

The integration of nanotechnology in liquid biofertilizers contributes to precision nutrient management.

3. **Integration of Artificial Intelligence (AI): Smart Farming Practices:**

   i. **AI-Driven Decision Support Systems:** Artificial Intelligence (AI) and machine learning algorithms can be harnessed to develop decision support systems for farmers. These systems can analyze diverse datasets, including soil health, weather conditions, crop characteristics, and historical performance, to provide personalized recommendations for the application of liquid biofertilizers. AI-driven insights enable farmers to make informed decisions and optimize their use of biofertilizers (Kumar, 2022).

   ii. **Remote Sensing Technologies:** Integration of remote sensing technologies, such as satellite imagery and unmanned aerial vehicles (UAVs), with AI algorithms enables real-time monitoring of crop health and nutrient status. This synergy facilitates the identification of areas in the field that may benefit from targeted applications of liquid biofertilizers, enhancing the precision and efficiency of nutrient management.

4. **Climate-Resilient Formulations: Adapting to Changing Environments:**

   i. **Drought-Tolerant Microorganisms:** With climate change leading to increased frequency and intensity of drought events, there is a growing need for biofertilizers that can thrive under water-stressed conditions. Research focused on identifying and engineering drought-tolerant microorganisms can contribute to the development of biofertilizers resilient to water scarcity.

   ii. **Biofertilizers for Climate-Adaptive Crops**: As agricultural systems adapt to changing climates, there is a need for biofertilizers tailored to the nutrient requirements of climate-adaptive crops. Developing formulations that align with the genetic traits and nutritional needs of climate-resilient crop varieties enhances the sustainability and productivity of agriculture in the face of climate variability.

5. **Circular Economy Approaches: Biofertilizer Production from Waste Streams:**

   i. **Utilization of Organic Waste:** Biofertilizers can be produced from organic waste streams, contributing to the circular economy. Microorganisms capable of nutrient solubilization and fixation can be employed to convert organic residues, such as agricultural and food processing waste, into valuable biofertilizer products. This approach not only addresses waste management challenges but also provides an eco-friendly source of nutrients.

   ii. **Symbiotic Microbe-Waste Interactions:** Investigating the symbiotic interactions between beneficial microorganisms and organic waste materials can uncover novel pathways for nutrient release. Understanding how microorganisms in biofertilizers interact with diverse organic substrates contributes to the development of sustainable and cost-effective waste-to-biofertilizer conversion processes.

6. **Multi-Strain Formulations: Harnessing Synergistic Effects:**

   i. **Synergistic Microbial Consortia:** Research focused on identifying and optimizing synergistic microbial consortia holds immense potential. Formulating biofertilizers with multiple strains of microorganisms that complement and enhance each.

4.6 CONCLUSION

In the pursuit of sustainable agriculture, liquid biofertilizers emerge as a beacon of promise and innovation. The journey through the intricate tapestry of microbial interactions, application techniques, and challenges underscores the transformative potential of biofertilizers in reshaping our approach to cultivation. At its core, the allure of liquid biofertilizers lies in their ability to redefine nutrient management. By tapping into the symbiotic relationships between microorganisms and plants, these biofertilizers offer a holistic alternative to conventional synthetic inputs. The synergistic dance of nitrogen-fixing bacteria, phosphorus-solubilizing microorganisms, and potassium-mobilizing agents not only enhances soil health but also mitigates environmental concerns associated with chemical fertilizers. This shift towards sustainable nutrient cycling aligns with the urgent need to preserve our ecosystems and promote resilient agricultural practices. Environmental stewardship takes center stage as liquid biofertilizers pave the way for reduced chemical dependency, mitigated soil and water pollution, and improved soil structure. The promise of cultivating in harmony with nature resonates in the environmental benefits, offering a pathway towards regenerative agriculture that nurtures both the land and the communities dependent on it. Economically, liquid biofertilizers prove to be a strategic investment, with cost-effectiveness, enhanced crop yields, and potential market access for sustainably produced crops. The social dimension of this agricultural transformation unfolds as small-scale farmers find empowerment through economic stability and improved livelihoods. The equitable distribution of benefits across farming communities amplifies the societal impact of biofertilizers, contributing to the broader goal of social equity in agriculture.

As technology propels us into the future, the trajectory of liquid biofertilizers aligns with the frontiers of innovation. Genetic engineering, nanotechnology, and AI usher in a new era of precision agriculture, where biofertilizers can be customized for specific crops and environmental conditions. This intersection of traditional wisdom and cutting-edge technology embodies the dynamic nature of sustainable agriculture, where adaptability and efficiency converge. In this ongoing journey, collaboration and education stand as cornerstones. Farmers, researchers, policymakers, and industry stakeholders must work hand in hand to bridge awareness gaps, dispel misconceptions, and pave the way for widespread adoption. As we conclude this exploration, the narrative of liquid biofertilizers for sustainable agriculture transcends the confines of a single solution—it encapsulates a vision for a future where cultivation is not just about yields but about fostering a resilient, regenerative, and harmonious relationship between humanity and the Earth.

KEYWORDS

- **biofertilizers**
- **cost-effectiveness**
- **cultivation**
- **drought-tolerant microorganisms**
- **microbe-waste interactions**
- **nutrient management**
- **sustainable agriculture**

REFERENCES

Ahirwar, N. K., Singh, R., Chaurasia, S., Chandra, R., & Ramana, S. (2020). Effective role of beneficial microbes in achieving the sustainable agriculture and eco-friendly environment development goals: A review. *Frontiers in Microbiology*, *5*, 111–123.

Allouzi, M. M. A., Allouzi, S. M. A., Keng, Z. X., Supramaniam, C. V., Singh, A., & Chong, S. (2022). Liquid biofertilizers as a sustainable solution for agriculture. *Helion.* https://www.cell.com/heliyon/home (accessed on 2nd January 2026).

Ammar, E. E., Rady, H. A., Khattab, A. M., Amer, M. H., Mohamed, S. A., Elodamy, N. I., & Aioub, A. A. (2023). A comprehensive overview of eco-friendly biofertilizers extracted from living organisms. *Environmental Science and Pollution Research, 30*(53), 113119–113137.

Arfarita, N., Lestari, M. W., & Prayogo, C. (2020). Utilization of vermiwash for the production of liquid biofertilizers and its effect on viability of inoculant bacteria and green bean germination. *AGRIVITA, Journal of Agricultural Science*, *42*(1), 120–130.

Asha, K., Krishna, H., Raju, K. K., & Guruprasad, V. (2023). Role of biofertilizers towards sustainable agricultural development: A review. *Journal of Advanced Applied Scientific Research*, *5*(5).

Çakmakçı, R. (2019). A review of biological fertilizers: Current use, new approaches, and future perspectives. *International Journal of Innovative Studies in Sciences and Engineering Technology*, *5*(7), 83–92.

Cha, B. K., Pandeya, B., Chanda, H., Bhusala, P., Pandita, S., & Khanalb, S. (2021). Promotion of organic and sustainable agriculture through the use of biofertilizers. *Journal of Wastes and Biomass Management (JWBM)*, *3*(1), 01–08.

Das, P., Khan, S., Chaudhary, A. K., AbdulQuadir, M., Thaher, M. I., & Al-Jabri, H. (2019). Potential applications of algae-based biofertilizer. In *Biofertilizers for Sustainable Agriculture and Environment* (pp. 41–65).

Dilnashin, H., Birla, H., Hoat, T. X., Singh, H. B., Singh, S. P., & Keswani, C. (2020). Applications of agriculturally important microorganisms for sustainable crop production.

In *Molecular Aspects of Plant Beneficial Microbes in Agriculture* (pp. 403–415). Academic Press.

Etesami, H., Emami, S., & Alikhani, H. A. (2017). Potassium solubilizing bacteria (KSB): Mechanisms, promotion of plant growth, and future prospects—A review. *Journal of Soil Science and Plant Nutrition, 17*(4), 897–911.

Gautam, K., Sirohi, C., Singh, N. R., Thakur, Y., Jatav, S. S., Rana, K., & Parihar, M. (2021). Microbial biofertilizer: Types, applications, and current challenges for sustainable agricultural production. In *Biofertilizers* (pp. 3–19). Woodhead Publishing.

Gul, A., Salam, A., Afridi, M. S., Bangash, N. K., Ali, F., Ali, M. Y., & Mubeeen, R. (2019). Effect of urea, biofertilizers and their interaction on the growth, yield and yield attributes of *Cyamopsis tetragonoloba. Indian Journal of Agricultural Research, 53*(4).

Gulshan, T., Verma, A., Ayoub, L., Sharma, J., Sharma, T., Bhadu, A., & Singh, B. (2022). Increasing nutrient use efficiency in crops through biofertilizers. https://www.researchgate.net/publication/363070237_Increasing_nutrient_use_efficiency_in_crops_through_biofertilizers (accessed on 2nd January 2026).

Handayani, T., Dewi, T. K., Martanti, D., Poerba, Y. S., Antonius, S., & Witjaksono, W. (2021). Application of inorganic and liquid organic biofertilizers affects the vegetative growth and rhizobacteria populations of eight banana cultivars. *Biodiverse Journal of Biological Diversity, 22*(3).

Jha, A., Pathania, D., Damathia, B., Raizada, P., Rustagi, S., Singh, P., & Chaudhary, V. (2023). Panorama of biogenic nano-fertilizers: A road to sustainable agriculture. *Environmental Research*, 116456.

Jin, K., Pezzuolo, A., Gouda, S. G., Jia, S., Eraky, M., Ran, Y., & Ai, P. (2022). Valorization of biofertilizer from anaerobic digestate through ammonia stripping process: A practical and sustainable approach towards circular economy. *Environmental Technology & Innovation, 27*, 102414.

Krishnaprabu, S. (2020). Liquid microbial consortium: A potential tool for sustainable soil health. *Journal of Pharmacognosy and Phytochemistry, 9*(2), 2191–2199.

Kumar, D., Dalal, R. P. S., & Arora, I. (2022). Biofertilizers: A future prospect towards sustainable agricultural development. In *Innovative Approaches for Sustainable Development: Theories and Practices in Agriculture* (pp. 91–105). Cham: Springer International Publishing.

Kumar, U. (2022, June). Biofertilizer technologies for enhancing nutrient use efficiency in rice. In *Souvenir, National Seminar on "Recent Developments in Nutrient Management Strategies for Sustainable Agriculture: The Indian Context* (p. 104).

Kumawat, H., Singh, D. P., Jat, G., Choudhary, R., Singh, P. B., Dhayal, S., & Khardia, N. (2021). Effect of fertility levels and liquid biofertilizers on growth and yield of wheat (*Triticum aestivum* L.). *The Pharma Innovation Journal, 10*(9), 1365–1369.

Kumawat, K. C., Nagpal, S., & Sharma, P. (2021). Present scenario of biofertilizer production and marketing around the globe. In *Biofertilizers* (pp. 389–413). Woodhead Publishing.

Meena, V. S., Parewa, H. P., Jeevan, B., Meena, S. K., & Meena, H. N. (2021). Liquid biofertilizer: A potential tool towards sustainable agriculture. *Soil Science: Fundamentals to Recent Advances*, 401–414.

Mohanty, N., Pattnaik, A. K., Mahapatra, P., Jena, N. K., Rout, S. K., & Ekka, M. S. (2021). Effect of macronutrients, biofertilizers and growth regulator on yield and yield attributing characters of capsicum (*Capsicum annuum* L.). *International Journal of Current Microbiology and Applied Sciences*, *10*(02), 2899–2906.

Mukherjee, B., Goswami, S., Pal, P., Mandal, T. K., Bhattacharya, U., Naskar, M. K., & Dutta, S. (2023). Improving crop nutrition through ecofriendly biofertilizers: Concept, types and benefits in agriculture.

Panda, D., Mondal, S., & Mishra, A. (2022). Liquid biofertilizers from seaweeds: A critical review. In *Sustainable Global Resources of Seaweeds Volume 1: Bioresources, Cultivation, Trade and Multifarious Applications* (pp. 485–501).

Patel, D., & Goswami, D. (2020). Phosphorus solubilization and mobilization: Mechanisms, current developments, and future challenge. In *Advances in Plant Microbiome and Sustainable Agriculture: Functional Annotation and Future Challenges* (pp. 1–20).

Peta, V. (2020). Utilizing rhizosphere and bacterial endophytes for use as potential biofertilizers for sustainable agricultural production. *South Dakota State University*.

Pogula, S. (2018). Biofertilizers and its importance in agriculture. *Indian Farmer*, 417.

Przygocka-Cyna, K., Barłóg, P., Spiżewski, T., & Grzebisz, W. (2021). Biofertilizers based on digestate and biomass ash as an alternative to commercial fertilizers—The case of tomato. *Agronomy*, *11*(9), 1716.

Sahu, S. K., Bindhani, S. K., Acharya, D., & Padhee, R. K. (2022). Development of nano biofertilizer via chemical & biological synthesis. *IRJMETS*, *4*(7), 1–17.

Satpute, A. V., Patil, J. B., Ghule, N. S., & Patil, M. J. (2021). Effect of inorganic and biofertilizers on yield attributes, yield and economic of summer groundnut *Arachis hypogaea* L. *International Journal of Chemical Studies*, *9*(1), 3289–3293.

Singh, J. S., Kumar, A., & Singh, M. (2019). Cyanobacteria: A sustainable and commercial bio-resource in production of biofertilizer and bio-fuel from waste waters. *Environmental and Sustainability Indicators*, *3*, 100008.

Singh, R., & Vyas, R. V. (2016). Innovative technologies and sustainable agricultural development. *Indian Research Journal of Extension Education*, *15*(3), 66–71.

Singh, S. P., Singh, S., Dubey, A. N., & Rajput, R. K. (2020). Biofertilizers and plant growth regulators as key player in sustainable agriculture by enhancing soil fertility and crop productivity. *Environment, Agriculture and Health*, *12*.

Tallou, A., Aziz, F., Garcia, A. J., Salcedo, F. P., El Minaoui, F. E., & Amir, S. (2021). Biofertilizers issued from anaerobic digestion for growing tomatoes under irrigation by treated wastewater: Targeting circular economy concept. *International Journal of Environmental Science and Technology*, 1–10.

Tyagi, S., Naresh, R. K., Prakash, S., Yadav, G., Tiwari, S., Rawat, B., & Sharma, N. (2019). Conservation agriculture, biofertilizers and biopesticides: A holistic approach for agricultural sustainability and food security: A review. *International Journal of Chemical Studies*, *7*, 3036–3046.

Upadhaya, B., Kaushal, K., & Kumar, R. (2022). Foxtail millet (*Setaria italica*) growth, yield and economics as affected by liquid biofertilizers and their mode of application. *The Pharma Innovation Journal*, *11*(2), 2225–2230.

Varshini, S. V., & Jayanthi, C. (2020). Organic liquid manures and biofertilizers: A tool for soil and crop productivity. *Agricultural Reviews*, *41*(4), 387–392.

Wable, N. B., & Khandelwal, R. K. (2023). Role of biofertilizers in sustainable agriculture development. *Disruptive Business Environment*, 421.

Yadav, K. K., & Sarkar, S. (2019). Biofertilizers, impact on soil fertility and crop productivity under sustainable agriculture. *Environment and Ecology*, *37*(1), 89–93.

Yadav, M. (2018). Biotechnology for sustainable agriculture and livelihood security: A preliminary review. *International Journal of Environmental Sciences*, *7*(2), 68–71.

Youssef, M. A., & Farag, M. I. H. (2021). Co-application of organic manure and biofertilizer to improve soil fertility and production of quinoa and proceeding Jew's mallow crops. *Journal of Soil Science and Plant Nutrition*, *21*(3), 2472–2488.

CHAPTER 5

Processing of Agri-Food Wastes: Role in Sustainable Agriculture

PRITI PAL,[1] PRAKASH KUMAR SARANGI,[2]
AKHILESH KUMAR SINGH,[3] ASHNA PARVEEN,[4] ANAND PRAKASH,[3]
BRIJESH PANDEY,[3] and UTTAM KUMAR SAHOO[5,*]

[1]*Amity Institute of Biotechnology, Amity University Uttar Pradesh, Lucknow Campus, Lucknow, India*

[2]*College of Agriculture, Central Agricultural University, Imphal, India*

[3]*Department of Biotechnology, School of Life Sciences, Mahatma Gandhi Central University, Motihari, Bihar, India*

[4]*Department of Biotechnology & Microbiology, Meerut Institute of Engineering and Technology, Baghpat Road Bypass Crossing, Meerut, India*

[5]*Department of Forestry, Mizoram University, Aizawl, India*

*Corresponding authors

ABSTRACT

Agri-food waste, a global challenge with significant environmental implications, is addressed through the lens of circular economy principles and innovative processing techniques. With approximately one-third of the world's food production lost or wasted, the environmental, economic, and social implications are significant. This chapter explores the application of circular economy principles, innovative processing techniques, and the resulting impact on soil health, economic diversification, and community engagement. The adoption of circular economy principles represents a

Biotechnology for Sustainable Agriculture: Innovative Approaches and Strategies.
Prakash Kumar Sarangi (Ed)

DOI: 10.1201/9781779642998-5

fundamental shift in waste management, emphasizing the need to transition from a linear model to a closed-loop system. The valorization of agri-food waste through recycling, reusing, and repurposing aligns with these principles, offering a sustainable solution to the global waste challenge. The creation of economic opportunities through the recovery of bioactive compounds, fertilizers, and energy products contributes to economic diversification, strengthening the resilience of agricultural systems. Despite the potential benefits, challenges in technological barriers, policy support, and public awareness persist. Overcoming these challenges requires investment in research, supportive policies, and public education campaigns to shift perceptions and actively engage stakeholders in waste reduction and valorization efforts.

5.1 INTRODUCTION

Agriculture, the cornerstone of global sustenance, confronts a paradoxical challenge as a substantial portion of the food produced is lost or wasted. In addressing this dilemma, the processing of agri-food waste emerges as a transformative force within the framework of sustainable agriculture. This chapter embarks on a comprehensive exploration of the intricacies surrounding agri-food waste, delving into circular economy principles, innovative processing techniques, and the multifaceted impacts on soil health, economic diversification, and community engagement (Ben-Othman et al., 2020). The global challenge of agri-food waste is staggering, with nearly one-third of the world's food production lost or wasted. Post-harvest losses, surplus production, and discarded by-products contribute to a complex web of environmental, economic, and societal implications. The urgency to mitigate this waste becomes apparent as the world grapples with a growing population and diminishing resources. Central to the transformation of waste management is the adoption of circular economy principles (Bhat, 2021). Departing from the traditional linear model of "take, make, dispose," a closed-loop system emerges where waste is not merely discarded but seen as a potential resource. The valorization of agri-food waste through recycling, reusing, and repurposing embodies the ethos of circularity, creating a sustainable feedback loop that minimizes waste and maximizes resource efficiency (Matei et al., 2021).

Processing techniques play a pivotal role in realizing the latent value within agri-food waste. Biological processes leverage microorganisms to convert organic waste into compost, biofuels, and organic fertilizers. Extraction techniques unearth bioactive compounds hidden within waste, with applications extending to pharmaceuticals, food, and cosmetics. Anaerobic digestion, a biological process converting organic waste into biogas and nutrient-rich digestate, emerges as a dual-purpose solution addressing energy needs and providing valuable fertilizers. Thermochemical processes, including pyrolysis and gasification, transform organic waste into biochar and syngas, offering solutions for both soil enhancement and energy production (Kassim et al., 2022).

The impact of waste processing extends profoundly to soil health and fertility. Organic amendments derived from processed waste, such as compost and biochar, transcend their origin as mere by-products to become instrumental in enhancing soil structure, water retention, and nutrient content. This symbiotic relationship between waste and soil health not only reduces the dependency on synthetic fertilizers but also cultivates a regenerative approach to agriculture (Papaioannou et al., 2022).

Economically, waste processing transcends the realm of waste management to economic diversification. The recovery of bioactive compounds, fertilizers, and energy products from agri-food waste creates novel revenue streams, fortifying the financial resilience of agricultural systems. Moreover, waste processing initiatives catalyze community engagement, generating employment opportunities and contributing to the socio-economic development of rural areas. This community involvement aligns with the ethos of sustainable agriculture, where empowerment and collective responsibility become integral. However, the journey towards waste processing is not without challenges. Technological barriers, policy imperatives, and the imperative for public awareness stand as hurdles that demand strategic navigation (Paini et al., 2022). Research investments, supportive policies, and comprehensive awareness campaigns become essential to overcoming these challenges and steering towards widespread adoption of sustainable waste management practices. Overall, the processing of agri-food waste emerges as a transformative force in reshaping the narrative of agriculture from a linear model of waste generation to a circular and regenerative approach. As we navigate the challenges of feeding a growing population within planetary boundaries, the role of waste processing becomes indispensable—a pathway to not only mitigate waste but to cultivate a sustainable, resilient, and empowered agricultural future. The integration of circular economy principles and innovative processing techniques paves the way for a holistic transformation of agri-food waste into a valuable resource, aligning with the broader goals of sustainability in agriculture (Smetana et al., 2018) (Figure 5.1).

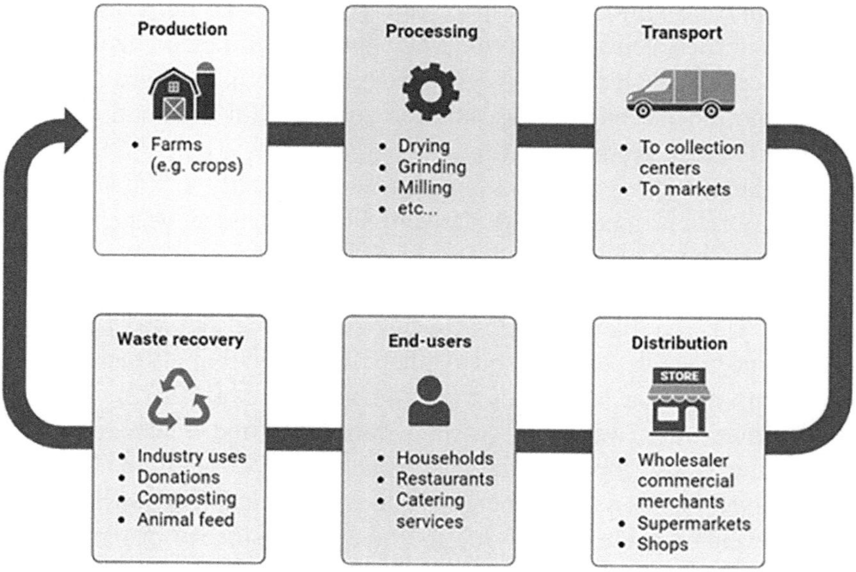

FIGURE 5.1 Progress in the production of food packaging using agricultural waste and by-products.

5.2 AGRI-FOOD WASTE: A GLOBAL CHALLENGE

The agricultural sector, while providing sustenance for a growing global population, grapples with a paradoxical dilemma—significant portions of the food produced are lost or wasted. This chapter delves into the intricate facets of agri-food waste as a pervasive global challenge, exploring the dimensions of post-harvest losses, surplus production, and discarded by-products that collectively contribute to nearly one-third of the world's food production being lost or wasted (Berenguer et al., 2022). The urgency to address this challenge stems from its profound environmental, economic, and social implications, making it a critical issue on the global agenda.

1. **The Magnitude of the Issue:** The sheer scale of agri-food waste is staggering. Post-harvest losses, resulting from inadequate storage, transportation, and handling, contribute significantly to

this challenge. Surplus production, driven by market demands and aesthetic standards, further exacerbates the issue. Additionally, the rejection of imperfect or surplus produce by consumers and retailers amplifies the volume of discarded food. The cumulative effect is a vast number of resources, including water, energy, and arable land, being squandered (Gebremikael et al., 2020).

2. **Environmental Consequences:** The environmental impact of agri-food waste is a cause for grave concern. The organic matter in decomposing food releases methane, a potent greenhouse gas that significantly contributes to climate change. Moreover, the extensive use of resources in the production of food that ultimately goes to waste intensifies pressure on ecosystems and exacerbates issues such as deforestation, water scarcity, and loss of biodiversity (Bhat, 2021). Addressing agri-food waste becomes pivotal in the context of mitigating climate change and promoting sustainable resource use.

3. **Economic Implications:** The economic ramifications of agri-food waste reverberate through the entire supply chain. Farmers incur losses due to unsold produce, and the economic value of resources invested in cultivating, harvesting, and transporting the wasted food is squandered. Retailers and distributors also suffer financial losses, leading to a less resilient and sustainable food supply chain. The economic impact extends beyond immediate financial losses, influencing food prices and market stability (Rodrigues et al., 2022).

4. **Social Dimensions:** At the societal level, the consequences of agri-food waste manifest in the stark contrast between abundance and scarcity. While a significant portion of the world's population faces hunger and malnutrition, edible food is discarded due to cosmetic imperfections or inefficiencies in the supply chain. Reducing agri-food waste is not only an economic imperative but also a moral and ethical obligation to ensure equitable access to food resources globally. Socially responsible practices in food production, distribution, and consumption become essential in addressing this dimension of the challenge (Kour et al., 2023).

5. **Food Security and Resource Scarcity**: The global challenge of agri-food waste intersects with the broader issues of food security

and resource scarcity. As the world population continues to grow, the demand for food surges, placing additional strain on already stressed resources. Efficient management of agri-food waste becomes instrumental in addressing the global food security conundrum, ensuring that available resources are utilized judiciously to meet the nutritional needs of a burgeoning population (Panzella et al., 2020).

6. **Changing Dietary Patterns**: Shifting dietary patterns contribute to the complexity of the agri-food waste challenge. As societies transition toward more resource-intensive diets, the environmental footprint of food production increases. The inefficiencies in the food supply chain become more pronounced when catering to the demands of meat-centric diets, leading to a disproportionate use of resources. Recognizing and addressing the impact of dietary choices on agri-food waste is integral to crafting sustainable solutions (Ciccullo et al., 2021).
7. **Technological and Infrastructural Disparities:** The challenge of agri-food waste is compounded by technological and infrastructural disparities across regions. Developed nations often have advanced technologies and robust infrastructure for storage, transportation, and processing, reducing the likelihood of post-harvest losses. In contrast, developing nations may lack these resources, leading to higher levels of waste at various stages of the supply chain (Chiaraluce et al., 2021). Bridging these disparities is essential for creating a more equitable and sustainable global food system.

5.3 CIRCULAR ECONOMY PRINCIPLES: NURTURING SUSTAINABILITY IN RESOURCE MANAGEMENT

Circular economy principles represent a departure from the linear economic model of "take, make, dispose" to a regenerative approach. This shift focuses on reusing, recycling, and repurposing resources to minimize waste and maximize efficiency. The principles are grounded in designing products for longevity and durability, ensuring they last and reduce the need for frequent replacements. Emphasis is placed on reusing and repurposing items to extend their lifecycles, reducing waste and conserving energy

(Chojnacka et al., 2022). Recycling and material recovery are integral to circular economy principles, aiming to extract value from products at the end of their life. Closing resource loops is a key goal, creating systems where materials are continually cycled. Product-as-a-service models encourage access over ownership, fostering product durability and ease of maintenance. Circular economy principles draw inspiration from nature, promoting biomimicry and nature-inspired design, where waste from one system becomes a resource for another (Konfo et al., 2023). Collaboration and stakeholder engagement are encouraged to optimize resource flows and share best practices. Digitalization and technology integration enhance the efficiency and transparency of circular systems. Regenerative agriculture practices align with circular principles, emphasizing soil health and closed nutrient cycles (Stillitano et al., 2021). The development of biomaterials from renewable resources contributes to circular manufacturing. Education and awareness play a crucial role in driving systemic change. A shift towards circularity requires an informed populace making sustainable choices. Circular economy principles provide a comprehensive framework for transitioning to a regenerative and sustainable economic model. By incorporating these principles into design, production, consumption, and waste management, societies can move towards a more resilient and environmentally responsible approach to resource management, crucial for mitigating environmental degradation and building a future that balances human well-being with ecological health (Szymczak et al., 2021).

5.3.1 PROCESSING TECHNIQUES FOR AGRI-FOOD WASTES

Processing techniques for agri-food wastes encompass a diverse array of methods aimed at converting these wastes into valuable resources, thereby addressing the challenges posed by waste accumulation in the agricultural sector (Romero-Perdomo et al., 2023). These techniques play a pivotal role in sustainable waste management, contributing to environmental conservation, resource efficiency, and the creation of secondary products that can be beneficial to various industries. Below, we elaborate on some key processing techniques for agri-food wastes:

1. **Biological Processes:**

   i. **Composting:** This is a natural and environmentally friendly method that utilizes microorganisms to decompose organic matter in agri-food wastes. This process results in nutrient-rich compost, a valuable soil conditioner and fertilizer (González-García et al., 2019).

ii. **Bioconversion:** Various microorganisms, such as bacteria and fungi, can be employed to bio convert agri-food wastes into biofuels, organic acids, and enzymes (González-García et al., 2019). This not only reduces waste volume but also generates products with potential industrial applications.

2. **Extraction of Bioactive Compounds:**

i. **Enzymatic Hydrolysis:** This technique involves using enzymes to break down complex organic molecules in agri-food wastes into simpler compounds. It is particularly useful for extracting bioactive compounds with applications in the pharmaceutical, food, and cosmetic industries (Bala et al., 2023).

ii. **Fermentation:** This utilizes microorganisms to break down organic matter in agri-food waste, producing bioactive compounds such as organic acids, vitamins, and antimicrobial agents (González-García et al., 2019).

3. **Anaerobic Digestion:** It is a biological process that occurs in the absence of oxygen. Microorganisms break down organic matter in agri-food wastes, producing biogas (mainly methane) and a nutrient-rich digestate. Biogas can be used for energy production, and the digestate can serve as an organic fertilizer (Sarkar et al., 2018).

4. **Thermochemical Processes:**

i. **Pyrolysis:** This involves heating agri-food waste in the absence of oxygen, leading to the decomposition of organic materials into biochar, syngas, and bio-oil. Biochar is a carbon-rich material that can enhance soil fertility, while syngas and bio-oil can be used for energy production (Priyadarshini and Abhilash, 2023).

ii. **Gasification:** Similar to pyrolysis, gasification transforms organic waste into syngas, which can be used for electricity generation or as a raw material for chemical synthesis (Tamburini et al., 2020).

5. **Mechanical Processes**

   i. **Mechanical Separation:** This involves using physical processes such as sieving, sorting, and screening to separate different components of agri-food waste. It is particularly useful for separating organic matter from non-biodegradable materials (Sangiorgio et al., 2022).

   ii. **Extrusion:** It is a mechanical process that involves forcing agri-food waste through a machine to produce a consistent product. It is often used in the production of feed pellets or biofuel briquettes (Sarkar et al., 2018).

6. **Supercritical Fluid Extraction (SFE):** This utilizes supercritical fluids, often carbon dioxide, to extract valuable compounds from agri-food waste. This technique is employed for extracting essential oils, flavors, and other high-value components (González-García et al., 2019).

7. **Electrochemical Processes:**

   i. **Electrochemical Oxidation:** Electrochemical processes involve the application of electrical energy to induce chemical reactions in agri-food waste. This can lead to the degradation of organic pollutants and the production of value-added chemicals.

These processing techniques highlight the versatility and innovation in transforming agri-food wastes into valuable resources. The choice of a specific technique often depends on the nature of the waste, the desired end-products, and the environmental and economic considerations associated with the processing method. Implementing these techniques not only helps manage waste but also contributes to the development of a more sustainable and circular agricultural system (Kusumowardani et al., 2022).

5.3.2 ROLE IN SOIL HEALTH AND FERTILITY

The processing of agri-food wastes plays a crucial role in enhancing soil health and fertility, offering a sustainable solution to soil management (Figure 5.2). The organic components derived from processed waste, such as compost and biochar, contribute to soil improvement through various mechanisms (Bhat and Jõudu, 2019). Below, we elaborate on the significant role of processed agri-food wastes in soil health and fertility:

1. **Organic Matter Addition:** Compost, a common product of agri-food waste processing, is rich in organic matter. When incorporated into the soil, organic matter improves soil structure, water retention, and nutrient-holding capacity. It serves as a source of energy for soil microorganisms, fostering microbial activity essential for nutrient cycling (Zarbà et al., 2021).

2. **Nutrient Enrichment:** Agri-food waste, after processing, contains essential nutrients such as nitrogen, phosphorus, and potassium. When incorporated into the soil, these nutrients become available to plants, promoting healthy growth and development. This nutrient enrichment reduces the need for synthetic fertilizers, contributing to sustainable agriculture (Chowdhary and Raj, 2023).

3. **Microbial Diversity and Activity:** The organic compounds in processed agri-food waste act as a substrate for soil microorganisms. This enhances microbial diversity and activity, crucial for nutrient mineralization and the breakdown of organic matter. Healthy microbial communities contribute to disease suppression, nutrient cycling, and overall soil resilience (Tanveer et al., 2021).

4. **pH Regulation:** Some processed agri-food waste products, such as biochar, have the ability to regulate soil pH. Biochar, a carbon-rich material derived from pyrolysis, can buffer soil acidity or alkalinity, creating an optimal pH range for plant growth. This is especially beneficial in soils with imbalances in pH levels (Mehmood et al., 2021).

5. **Improved Water Retention:** The addition of processed agri-food waste, particularly compost, enhances soil water retention capacity. The organic matter acts like a sponge, holding water and reducing the risk of water runoff (Mehmood et al., 2021). This is vital for plant water uptake, especially in regions prone to drought or erratic precipitation patterns.

6. **Reduction in Soil Erosion:** The improvement in soil structure resulting from the addition of processed agri-food waste helps

mitigate soil erosion. Enhanced soil aggregation reduces surface runoff, preventing the loss of topsoil and preserving the integrity of the soil profile (Chiaraluce, 2021).

7. **Carbon Sequestration:** Biochar, a by-product of thermo-chemical processes, contributes to carbon sequestration. When applied to the soil, biochar acts as a stable form of organic carbon, sequestering carbon in the soil for an extended period. This helps mitigate climate change by reducing atmospheric carbon dioxide levels (Czekała et al., 2022).

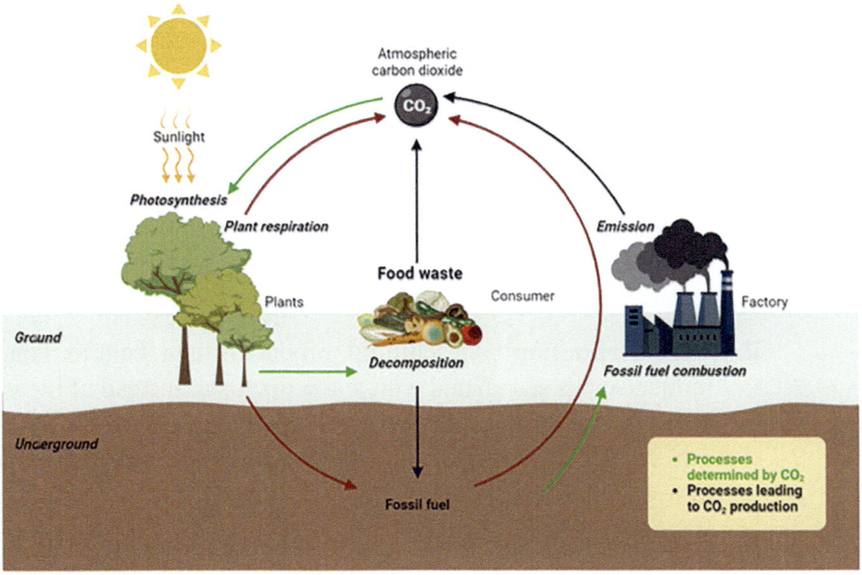

FIGURE 5.2 Crops for carbon farming.

8. **Enhanced Soil Biodiversity:** The presence of organic matter from processed agri-food waste provides a habitat and food source for diverse soil organisms. Increased soil biodiversity, including beneficial insects, earthworms, and microbial communities, contributes to a more resilient and ecologically balanced soil ecosystem (Facchini et al., 2022).

9. **Reduction of Environmental Impact:** By recycling agri-food waste into valuable soil amendments, the environmental impact

of waste disposal is minimized. This practice aligns with the principles of a circular economy, where waste is converted into a resource, fostering sustainable and responsible agricultural practices (Molina et al., 2023).

5.3.3 ECONOMIC AND SOCIAL DIMENSIONS

The processing of agri-food wastes holds substantial economic and social dimensions, contributing to the creation of a more sustainable and resilient agricultural system (Visco et al., 2022). Below, we elaborate on the economic and social aspects associated with the processing of agri-food wastes:

1. **Economic Dimensions:**

   i. **Revenue Generation:** The processing of agri-food wastes leads to the creation of valuable products such as compost, biofuels, and bioactive compounds. These products can be commercialized, creating new revenue streams for farmers, waste management industries, and entrepreneurs engaged in waste processing ventures.

   ii. **Cost Reduction:** Agricultural producers can benefit from reduced costs associated with waste disposal. Instead of incurring expenses for waste removal, processing agri-food waste into valuable products can offset disposal costs and contribute to overall farm profitability.

   iii. **Resource Efficiency:** The reuse of processed agri-food waste as organic fertilizers or soil amendments reduces the need for synthetic fertilizers. This enhances resource efficiency, as the nutrients in the waste are recycled back into the agricultural system, minimizing the reliance on external inputs.

   iv. **Job Creation:** Establishing and operating facilities for the processing of agri-food waste can generate employment opportunities. From waste collection and transportation to processing and distribution, the entire value chain creates jobs, particularly in rural areas where agriculture is a significant economic driver.

v. **Diversification of Income Sources:** The creation of value-added products from processed agri-food waste allows farmers and businesses to diversify their income sources. Revenue generated from waste-derived products can act as a supplementary income, reducing dependency on income solely derived from traditional agricultural practices.

vi. **Market Opportunities:** Processed agri-food waste, such as bioactive compounds extracted from waste streams, can tap into markets beyond traditional agriculture. These compounds have applications in pharmaceuticals, cosmetics, and food industries, opening up new market opportunities and potentially contributing to export revenues.

2. **Social Dimensions:**

i. **Community Engagement:** Localized waste processing initiatives foster community engagement. When communities are involved in waste management practices, there is a sense of ownership and responsibility. This engagement can lead to the establishment of community-based processing facilities, creating a shared commitment to sustainable practices.

ii. **Socio-Economic Development:** Waste processing initiatives contribute to socio-economic development in rural areas. The creation of jobs and income-generating activities associated with waste processing enhances the economic resilience of communities, potentially lifting them out of poverty and improving overall well-being (Papaioannou et al., 2022).

iii. **Public Awareness and Education:** The processing of agri-food wastes provides opportunities for public awareness and education. Initiatives focused on waste reduction, recycling, and sustainable agricultural practices can enhance public understanding of the environmental impact of waste and the importance of responsible waste management.

iv. **Environmental Stewardship:** The social dimension of waste processing is closely tied to environmental stewardship. When communities actively participate in waste reduction and recycling efforts, there is a collective contribution to environmental preservation. This sense of responsibility for the environment fosters a culture of sustainability.

v. **Health and Quality of Life:** Proper waste management, including the processing of agri-food waste, contributes to a healthier living environment. Reduced waste pollution positively impacts air and water quality, enhancing the overall health and quality of life for communities residing in agricultural areas.

vi. **Empowerment of Local Producers:** The utilization of agri-food waste for local production, such as compost for community gardens or bioenergy for local power generation, empowers local producers. This decentralized approach to waste utilization contributes to self-sufficiency and resilience at the community level.

5.3.4 CHALLENGES IN THE PROCESSING OF AGRI-FOOD WASTES

1. **Technological Barriers:** Many processing techniques for agri-food wastes require specialized technologies, and small-scale or resource-constrained agricultural settings may face challenges in adopting these advanced methods.

2. **Infrastructure Limitations:** In some regions, especially in developing countries, inadequate infrastructure for waste collection, transportation, and processing poses significant challenges. The lack of proper facilities hinders the efficient implementation of waste processing initiatives.

3. **Policy and Regulatory Frameworks:** Inconsistent or unclear policies and regulations related to waste processing can impede progress. Harmonizing policies and creating supportive regulatory frameworks are crucial for the widespread adoption of sustainable waste management practices.

4. **Public Awareness and Participation:** Limited public awareness about the benefits of waste processing and recycling can hinder community participation. Education and outreach programs are essential to inform and engage the public in responsible waste management practices.

5. **Financial Constraints:** Establishing and maintaining waste processing facilities require initial investments and ongoing operational costs. Financial constraints, particularly for small farmers or businesses, may limit their ability to implement waste processing initiatives.

6. **Market Demand for Products:** The market demand for products derived from processed agri-food waste, such as compost or bio-based materials, may vary. Ensuring a stable market for these products is essential for the economic viability of waste processing ventures (Chen et al., 2018).

7. **Contamination Issues:** Contamination of agri-food waste streams with non-biodegradable materials, such as plastics or heavy metals, poses challenges for processing. Separating and managing contaminants can be technically challenging and financially burdensome.

8. **Scale-Up Challenges:** Successful waste processing initiatives at a small scale may encounter challenges when scaling up. Issues related to logistics, technology adaptation, and resource availability need to be carefully addressed during the scaling-up process.

5.4 FUTURE PERSPECTIVES AND RESEARCH DIRECTIONS

1. **Advanced Technologies:** Continued research into advanced processing technologies, including more efficient biological and thermochemical methods, can enhance the effectiveness of agri-food waste conversion while addressing scalability and cost challenges.

2. **Decentralized Processing Models:** Exploring decentralized waste processing models, especially in rural areas, can overcome infrastructure limitations. Mobile or community-based processing units may offer a flexible and adaptive approach to waste management.

3. **Circular Economy Integration:** Integrate waste processing into a broader circular economy framework, emphasizing the development of closed-loop systems where waste becomes a resource.

This approach maximizes resource efficiency and minimizes environmental impact (Gebremikael et al., 2020).

4. **Policy Reforms:** Advocate for policy reforms that support sustainable waste management practices. This includes incentivizing waste processing initiatives, establishing clear regulations, and creating a conducive environment for investment in waste-to-value ventures.

5. **Technological Innovation for Contaminant Removal:** Invest in research to develop technologies capable of efficiently removing contaminants from agri-food waste streams. Innovative methods for separation and purification can improve the quality of processed waste products (Adegbeye et al., 2020).

6. **Market Development:** Work towards creating stable and diverse markets for products derived from agri-food waste. Encouraging industries to adopt sustainable practices and promoting consumer awareness can drive demand for these products (Mangla et al., 2018).

7. **Cross-Sectoral Collaboration:** Encourage collaboration between agricultural, environmental, and industrial sectors to create synergies in waste processing. Collaborative efforts can lead to holistic solutions that address waste challenges at various stages of the supply chain.

8. **Education and Outreach:** Invest in educational programs to raise awareness about the environmental and economic benefits of waste processing. Outreach initiatives targeting farmers, businesses, and the general public can promote a culture of responsible waste management.

9. **Investment in Research and Development:** Allocate resources for ongoing research and development to explore new and improved waste processing technologies. This includes understanding the potential of emerging technologies and adapting them to the specific needs of diverse agricultural systems (Rejeb et al., 2021).

5.5 CLIMATE CHANGE MITIGATION

Recognize the role of waste processing in climate change mitigation. Position waste management as a key component of strategies to reduce greenhouse gas emissions, promote carbon sequestration, and contribute to overall climate resilience.

Addressing the challenges and exploring future perspectives in the processing of agri-food wastes requires a collaborative effort involving researchers, policymakers, industries, and communities. By overcoming these challenges and advancing research in key areas, the potential for creating a sustainable and circular agricultural system becomes increasingly achievable (Borrello et al., 2016).

5.6 CONCLUSION

In conclusion, the processing of agri-food wastes emerges as a pivotal player in the journey toward sustainable agriculture, offering multifaceted benefits that extend far beyond waste reduction. This chapter has delved into the intricate web of challenges, opportunities, and transformative impacts associated with the responsible management of agricultural residues. From biological processes like composting to advanced technologies such as pyrolysis, each processing technique contributes to reshaping the narrative of waste from a burden to a valuable resource. The economic dimensions of waste processing are profound, with the creation of new revenue streams, cost reductions, and job opportunities. As processed waste transforms into valuable products like compost, biofuels, and bioactive compounds, it not only offsets disposal costs but also contributes to the economic resilience of agricultural communities. The diversification of income sources and the opening of new market opportunities underscore the potential of waste processing as an economic catalyst within the agricultural sector.

Simultaneously, the social dimensions echo a narrative of community engagement, socio-economic development, and environmental stewardship. The creation of jobs, especially in rural areas, empowers communities and enhances overall well-being. Public awareness campaigns and educational initiatives foster a culture of responsibility, instilling an understanding of the environmental impact of waste and the importance of sustainable waste management practices. This collective sense of responsibility for the environment contributes to a healthier and more vibrant living environment. The role of processed agri-food waste in soil health and fertility further solidifies its significance. From organic matter addition and nutrient enrichment to microbial diversity enhancement, the processed waste becomes an instrumental player in cultivating resilient and productive soils. These improvements, in turn, contribute to sustainable agriculture by reducing the dependence on synthetic fertilizers, mitigating soil erosion, and promoting water retention. However, the journey toward fully realizing the potential of waste processing is not without its challenges. Technological barriers, infrastructure limitations, and policy inconsistencies present hurdles that demand strategic navigation. Overcoming these challenges requires collaborative efforts, investment in research and development, and the formulation of supportive policy frameworks. The future perspectives outlined suggest a pathway forward that involves advanced technologies, decentralized processing models, and circular economy integration.

In essence, the processing of agri-food wastes transcends the traditional linear model of waste disposal, ushering in an era of circularity, resource efficiency, and sustainability. As waste becomes a valuable resource, agriculture evolves into a more resilient and regenerative system. The holistic integration of waste processing into agricultural practices not only addresses immediate waste challenges but also contributes to broader goals of environmental conservation, economic prosperity, and community well-being. In the journey towards sustainable agriculture, waste processing stands as a beacon, guiding the way to a future where agricultural systems thrive in harmony with the environment.

KEYWORDS

- **agricultural practices**
- **agri-food wastes**
- **economic dimensions**
- **policy frameworks**
- **socio-economic development**
- **soil erosion**
- **synthetic fertilizers**

REFERENCES

Adegbeye, M. J., Reddy, P. R. K., Obaisi, A. I., Elghandour, M. M. M. Y., Oyebamiji, K. J., Salem, A. Z. M., & Camacho-Díaz, L. M. (2020). Sustainable agriculture options for production, greenhouse gasses and pollution alleviation, and nutrient recycling in emerging and transitional nations—An overview. *Journal of Cleaner Production, 242*, 118319.

Bala, S., Garg, D., Sridhar, K., Inbaraj, B. S., Singh, R., Kamma, S., & Sharma, M. (2023). Transformation of agro-waste into value-added bioproducts and bioactive compounds: Micro/nano formulations and application in the agri-food-pharma sector. *Bioengineering, 10*(2), 152.

Ben-Othman, S., Jõudu, I., & Bhat, R. (2020). Bioactive from agri-food wastes: Present insights and future challenges. *Molecules, 25*(3), 510.

Berenguer, C. V., Andrade, C., Pereira, J. A., Perestrelo, R., & Câmara, J. S. (2022). Current challenges in the sustainable valorization of agri-food wastes: A review. *Processes, 11*(1), 20.

Bhat, R. (2021). Sustainability challenges in the valorization of agri-food wastes and by-products. In *Valorization of Agri-Food Wastes and By-Products* (pp. 1–27). Academic Press.

Bhat, R. (2021). *Valorization of Agri-Food Wastes and By-Products: Recent Trends, Innovations and Sustainability Challenges.*

Bhat, R., & Jõudu, I. (2019). Emerging issues and challenges in agri-food supply chain. In *Sustainable Food Supply Chains* (pp. 23–37).

Borrello, M., Lombardi, A., Pascucci, S., & Cembalo, L. (2016). The seven challenges for transitioning into a bio-based circular economy in the agri-food sector. *Recent Patents on Food, Nutrition & Agriculture, 8*(1), 39–47.

Chen, H., Liu, S., Zhao, G., Oderanti, F., Guyon, C., & Boshkoska, B. M. (2018). Identifying knowledge brokers, artefacts and channels for waste reduction in agri-food supply chains. *International Journal of Sustainable Agricultural Management and Informatics, 4*(3–4), 273–289.

Chiaraluce, G. (2021). Circular economy in the agri-food sector: A policy overview. *Italian Review of Agricultural Economics, 76*(3), 53–60.

Chiaraluce, G., Bentivoglio, D., & Finco, A. (2021). Circular economy for a sustainable agri-food supply chain: A review for current trends and future pathways. *Sustainability, 13*(16), 9294.

Chojnacka, K., Moustakas, K., & Mikulewicz, M. (2022). Valorization of agri-food waste to fertilizers is a challenge in implementing the circular economy concept in practice. *Environmental Pollution, 312*, 119906.

Chowdhary, P., & Raj, A. (2023). *Agri-Food Waste Valorization.* Royal Society of Chemistry.

Ciccullo, F., Cagliano, R., Bartezzaghi, G., & Perego, A. (2021). Implementing the circular economy paradigm in the agri-food supply chain: The role of food waste prevention technologies. *Resources, Conservation and Recycling, 164*, 105114.

Czekała, W., Janczak, D., Pochwatka, P., Nowak, M., & Dach, J. (2022). Gases emissions during composting process of agri-food industry waste. *Applied Sciences, 12*(18), 9245.

Facchini, F., Silvestri, B., Digiesi, S., & Lucchese, A. (2022). Agri-food loss and waste management: Win-win strategies for edible discarded fruits and vegetables sustainable reuse. *Innovative Food Science & Emerging Technologies*, 103235.

Gebremikael, M. T., Ranasinghe, A., Hosseini, P. S., Laboan, B., Sonneveld, E., Pipan, M., & De Neve, S. (2020). How do novel and conventional agri-food wastes, co-products and by-products improve soil functions and soil quality? *Waste Management, 113*, 132–144.

González-García, S., Gullón, P., & Gullón, B. (2019). Bio-compounds production from agri-food wastes under a biorefinery approach: Exploring environmental and social sustainability. In *Quantification of Sustainability Indicators in the Food Sector* (pp. 25–53).

Kassim, F. O., Thomas, C. P., & Afolabi, O. O. (2022). Integrated conversion technologies for sustainable agri-food waste valorization: A critical review. *Biomass and Bioenergy, 156*, 106314.

Konfo, T. R. C., Djouhou, F. M. C., Hounhouigan, M. H., Dahouenon-Ahoussi, E., Avlessi, F., & Sohounhloue, C. K. D. (2023). Recent advances in the use of digital technologies in agri-food processing: A short review. *Applied Food Research*, 100329.

Kour, R., Singh, S., Sharma, H. B., Naik, T. S. S. K., Shehata, N., Pavithra, N., & Ramamurthy, P. C. (2023). Persistence and remote sensing of agri-food wastes in the environment: Current state and perspectives. *Chemosphere*, 137822.

Kusumowardani, N., Tjahjono, B., Lazell, J., Bek, D., Theodorakopoulos, N., Andrikopoulos, P., & Priadi, C. R. (2022). A circular capability framework to address food waste and losses in the agri-food supply chain: The antecedents, principles and outcomes of circular economy. *Journal of Business Research, 142*, 17–31.

Mangla, S. K., Luthra, S., Rich, N., Kumar, D., Rana, N. P., & Dwivedi, Y. K. (2018). Enablers to implement sustainable initiatives in agri-food supply chains. *International Journal of Production Economics, 203*, 379–393.

Matei, E., Râpă, M., Predescu, A. M., Țurcanu, A. A., Vidu, R., Predescu, C., & Orbeci, C. (2021). Valorization of agri-food wastes as sustainable eco-materials for wastewater treatment: Current state and new perspectives. *Materials, 14*(16), 4581.

Mehmood, A., Ahmed, S., Viza, E., Bogush, A., & Ayyub, R. M. (2021). Drivers and barriers towards circular economy in agri-food supply chain: A review. *Business Strategy & Development, 4*(4), 465–481.

Molina, G., Sharma, M., Benhida, R., Gupta, V. K., & Kuhad, R. C. (2023). *Microbial Bioprocessing of Agri-Food Wastes: Bioactive Molecules*. CRC Press.

Paini, J., Benedetti, V., Ail, S. S., Castaldi, M. J., Baratieri, M., & Patuzzi, F. (2022). Valorization of wastes from the food production industry: A review towards an integrated agri-food processing biorefinery. *Waste and Biomass Valorization*, 1–20.

Panzella, L., Moccia, F., Nasti, R., Marzorati, S., Verotta, L., & Napolitano, A. (2020). Bioactive phenolic compounds from agri-food wastes: An update on green and sustainable extraction methodologies. *Frontiers in Nutrition, 7*, 60.

Papaioannou, E. H., Mazzei, R., Bazzarelli, F., Piacentini, E., Giannakopoulos, V., Roberts, M. R., & Giorno, L. (2022). Agri-food industry waste as resource of chemicals: The role of membrane technology in their sustainable recycling. *Sustainability, 14*(3), 1483.

Priyadarshini, P., & Abhilash, P. C. (2023). An empirical analysis of resource efficiency and circularity within the agri-food sector of India. *Journal of Cleaner Production, 385*, 135660.

Rejeb, A., Rejeb, K., & Zailani, S. (2021). Big data for sustainable agri-food supply chains: A review and future research perspectives. *Journal of Data, Information and Management, 3*, 167–182.

Rodrigues, J. P., Liberal, Â., Petropoulos, S. A., Ferreira, I. C., Oliveira, M. B. P., Fernandes, Â., & Barros, L. (2022). Agri-food surplus, waste and loss as sustainable biobased ingredients: A review. *Molecules, 27*(16), 5200.

Romero-Perdomo, F., & González-Curbelo, M. Á. (2023). Integrating multi-criteria techniques in life-cycle tools for the circular bioeconomy transition of agri-food waste biomass: A systematic review. *Sustainability, 15*(6), 5026.

Sangiorgio, P., Verardi, A., Dimatteo, S., Spagnoletta, A., Moliterni, S., & Errico, S. (2022). Valorization of agri-food waste and mealworms rearing residues for improving the sustainability of *Tenebrio molitor* industrial production. *Journal of Insects as Food and Feed, 8*(5), 509–524.

Sarkar, S. F., Poon, J. S., Lepage, E., Bilecki, L., & Girard, B. (2018). Enabling a sustainable and prosperous future through science and innovation in the bioeconomy at Agriculture and Agri-Food Canada. *New Biotechnology, 40*, 70–75.

Smetana, S., Aganovic, K., Irmscher, S., & Heinz, V. (2018). Agri-food waste streams utilization for development of more sustainable food substitutes. In *Designing Sustainable Technologies, Products and Policies: From Science to Innovation* (pp. 145–155).

Stillitano, T., Spada, E., Iofrida, N., Falcone, G., & De Luca, A. I. (2021). Sustainable agri-food processes and circular economy pathways in a life cycle perspective: State of the art of applicative research. *Sustainability, 13*(5), 2472.

Szymczak, T., Cybulska, J., Podleśny, M., & Frąc, M. (2021). Various perspectives on microbial lipase production using agri-food waste and renewable products. *Agriculture, 11*(6), 540.

Tamburini, E., Gaglio, M., Castaldelli, G., & Fano, E. A. (2020). Biogas from agri-food and agricultural waste can appreciate agro-ecosystem services: The case study of Emilia Romagna region. *Sustainability, 12*(20), 8392.

Tanveer, U., Ishaq, S., & Gough, A. (2021). Circular economy in agri-food sector: Food waste management perspective. In *Challenges and Opportunities of Circular Economy in Agri-Food Sector: Rethinking Waste* (pp. 55–75).

Visco, A., Scolaro, C., Facchin, M., Brahimi, S., Belhamdi, H., Gatto, V., & Beghetto, V. (2022). Agri-food wastes for bioplastics: European prospective on possible applications in their second life for a circular economy. *Polymers, 14*(13), 2752.

Zarbà, C., Chinnici, G., La Via, G., Bracco, S., Pecorino, B., & D'Amico, M. (2021). Regulatory elements on the circular economy: Driving into the agri-food system. *Sustainability, 13*(15), 8350.

CHAPTER 6

Beneficial Microbes for Management of Insects: Role in Sustainable Agriculture

PRITI PAL,[1] PRAKASH KUMAR SARANGI,[2]
AKHILESH KUMAR SINGH,[3] AHMAD GAZALI,[3]
UTTAM KUMAR SAHOO,[4] BRIJESH PANDEY,[3] and
ANAND PRAKASH[3,*]

[1]*Amity Institute of Biotechnology, Amity University Uttar Pradesh, Lucknow Campus, Lucknow, India*

[2]*College of Agriculture, Central Agricultural University, Imphal, Manipur, India*

[3]*Department of Biotechnology, School of Life Sciences, Mahatma Gandhi Central University, Motihari, Bihar, India*

[4]*Department of Forestry, Mizoram University, Aizawl, Mizoram, India*

*Corresponding authors

ABSTRACT

Beneficial microbes offer a diversified toolbox for insect management, ranging from direct effects, such as pathogenicity and parasitism, to indirect mechanisms like plant-mediated defenses and systemic resistance. Case studies exemplify successful microbial pest control, demonstrating their practical application in agriculture. Despite their potential, challenges in application, safety considerations, and comparisons with chemical pesticides underscore the need for a nuanced approach. The abstract navigates the intricate tripartite interactions among plants, microbes, and insects, exploring induced systemic resistance and the manipulation of plant volatiles. Integration into integrated pest management (IPM) strategies

Biotechnology for Sustainable Agriculture: Innovative Approaches and Strategies.
Prakash Kumar Sarangi (Ed)

DOI: 10.1201/9781779642998-6

emphasizes synergies with other control methods and strategic applications. Environmental and ecological considerations, including impacts on non-target organisms and regulatory frameworks, are crucial in assessing the overall sustainability of microbial approaches. As agriculture looks to the future, these abstract highlights the transformative potential of beneficial microbes, encouraging ongoing research into advanced technologies, novel strains, and collaborative efforts. The utilization of these microbes presents a dynamic pathway toward a more resilient and environmentally conscious agricultural future.

6.1 INTRODUCTION

In the vast tapestry of agriculture, the perennial struggle against insect pests has been a persistent challenge, demanding innovative solutions that align with the evolving ethos of sustainable practices. The realization that traditional pest control measures, often reliant on chemical pesticides, can be environmentally detrimental has prompted a paradigm shift. Enter the realm of beneficial microbes, a burgeoning frontier in integrated pest management (IPM) that holds the promise of revolutionizing how we navigate the delicate balance between productivity and ecological harmony in agriculture (Ahirwar et al., 2020). The quest for sustainable agriculture is not merely an ideological pursuit but a pragmatic response to the pressing challenges posed by conventional pest management. Over the years, the widespread use of chemical pesticides has not only raised concerns about environmental contamination but has also given rise to issues such as pesticide resistance, ecological imbalances, and unintended harm to non-target organisms. It is within this backdrop that the role of beneficial microbes gains prominence as a compelling alternative, offering a nuanced and ecologically harmonious approach to insect management (Thakur et al., 2020). Beneficial microbes encompass an array of microscopic organisms that include bacteria, fungi, and viruses, each wielding unique capabilities that can be harnessed for pest control. The narrative of their utilization unfolds as a chronicle of natural allies coaxed into service, a strategic alliance with the microbial world that dates back to ancient agricultural practices. As we embark on this exploration, it is imperative to delve into the foundational understanding of beneficial microbes, unraveling their diversity, functions, and the intricate ways in which they engage with both plants and insects (Elnahal et al., 2022). The sheer diversity within the microbial realm is staggering, each microorganism a potential soldier in the battle against agricultural pests. Bacteria, such as *Bacillus thuringiensis* (*Bt*), have long been recognized for their insecticidal properties, while fungi like *Beauveria bassiana* wield their pathogenic prowess against a spectrum of insects. Viruses too, in the form of baculoviruses, emerge as formidable contenders in this microbial orchestra, each with its own set of mechanisms that can be exploited for precise and targeted insect control (Ortiz and Sansinenea, 2022).

The historical tapestry of agriculture is woven with threads of microbial influence. Before the advent of synthetic pesticides, farmers relied on the natural predilections of beneficial microbes to curb pest populations. The renaissance of this age-old practice in contemporary agriculture is not merely a return to antiquity but a convergence of ancient wisdom with modern scientific understanding. Beneficial microbes, once consigned to the margins of traditional knowledge, are now taking center stage in the ongoing narrative of sustainable agriculture (Qadri et al., 2020). The nuanced dance between beneficial microbes, plants, and insects unfolds in a narrative that spans direct and indirect modes of interaction. The direct mechanisms involve the microorganisms acting as pathogens or parasites, directly impacting the physiology and life cycle of the target insect pests. Indirect interactions, on the other hand, encompass a more intricate ballet where the microorganisms influence the plant's physiology, inducing systemic resistance and arming the plants with innate capabilities to defend against insect invasions. Case studies dot this landscape, showcasing instances where the strategic deployment of beneficial microbes has translated theory into tangible success stories in the field. These microorganisms, once relegated to the role of biological curiosities, are now recognized as powerful agents of change, capable of reshaping the ecological dynamics of agricultural landscapes (Naik et al., 2019). These case studies not only underscore the practicality of microbial pest control but also reveal the complexities and challenges inherent in the application of these strategies on a larger scale. Yet, the journey towards embracing beneficial microbes in agriculture is not devoid of challenges. It is a nuanced path, navigating the intricacies of microbial behavior, the potential for unintended consequences, and the realities of on-the-ground application. The road is dotted with considerations of safety, efficacy, and the adaptability of these microbial allies in diverse agroecosystems. As agriculture embraces a more sustainable trajectory, it does so with a pragmatic acknowledgment of the complexities that accompany this microbial revolution (Ray et al., 2020).

In the arena of microbial pest control, bacteria take center stage, notably *Bacillus thuringiensis* (*Bt*). This microbial warrior has been a stalwart ally in the fight against insect pests, producing toxins lethal to specific insect groups. The versatility of *Bt*, coupled with its environmentally friendly profile, positions it as a cornerstone in microbial pest control strategies. Bacterial insecticides, including various strains of *Bt*, have found their niche in organic farming and IPM programs, carving a path towards more ecologically harmonious agriculture. Fungi, too, emerge as formidable players in the microbial orchestra of insect management (Olaniyan and Adetunji, 2021). Among them, *Beauveria bassiana* stands out as a versatile entomopathogenic fungus, capable of infecting a wide range of insect hosts. Its mode of action, involving attachment to the insect cuticle and subsequent penetration, showcases the intricacies of microbial warfare at the microscopic level. The environmentally benign nature of these fungal biopesticides positions them as potent tools in sustainable agriculture, offering a targeted and species-specific approach to pest control. The narrative extends to the viral realm, where baculoviruses take center stage. These viruses, with their unique specificity to certain insect species, are employed as bioinsecticides, posing minimal risk to non-target organisms (Trivedi et al., 2021). The viral biopesticides exemplify the precision that can be achieved through microbial strategies, targeting only the intended insect pests while leaving beneficial insects unharmed. However, the story of beneficial microbes extends beyond the microbial arsenal against pests. It encompasses a complex web of interactions that involves plants as active participants in this ecological drama. Microbes become architects of plant defenses, inducing systemic resistance and priming plants to respond more effectively to insect attacks. This plant-mediated defense mechanism represents a paradigm shift, transforming plants from passive victims to active participants in the ongoing struggle against insect pests (Ruiu, 2020). Induced systemic resistance (ISR) is a phenomenon where plants, primed by beneficial microbes, exhibit enhanced resistance to a broad spectrum of pathogens, including insects. This transformation at the plant level involves complex signaling pathways, where the presence of certain microbes triggers a cascade of events that culminate in a heightened state of alertness against potential threats. It is a remarkable example of the intricate ways in which the plant and microbial worlds converge, creating a synergistic defense mechanism that transcends the boundaries of individual organisms. Microbes, in their alliance with plants, also play a role in shaping the volatile compounds released by plants (Rai et al., 2020). These plant volatiles, once considered mere fragrances, are revealed as essential components of a sophisticated communication system between plants and insects. Beneficial microbes influence the emission of these volatiles, creating an aromatic arsenal that can either repel insect pests or attract their natural enemies. This orchestration of volatile compounds becomes a subtle yet powerful tool in the hands of microbial allies, transforming the very air around plants into a medium of ecological communication (O'Callaghan et al., 2022).

As agriculture stands at the intersection of tradition and innovation, the integration of beneficial microbes into broader pest management strategies becomes increasingly pivotal. IPM approaches, which seek to combine multiple strategies for effective pest control, find a natural ally in beneficial microbes. The synergies between microbial strategies and other control methods, such as cultural practices and the judicious use of synthetic pesticides, represent a holistic approach to pest management. It is a departure from the singular reliance on chemical interventions, marking a transition towards a more integrated and sustainable agricultural paradigm. The integration of beneficial microbes into IPM is not merely a tactical maneuver but a strategic shift in the way we conceptualize and implement pest management. It demands a nuanced understanding of the ecological intricacies at play, considering not only the immediate impact on pest populations but also the long-term implications for agroecosystem health (Rastegari et al., 2020). This integrated approach acknowledges the complexity of agricultural landscapes, where diverse factors, from climatic conditions to the presence of natural enemies, influence the dynamics of pest populations.

However, the application of beneficial microbes in the field is not without its challenges. The translational journey from laboratory success to on-the-ground efficacy involves navigating a terrain fraught with complexities. Issues of scalability, adaptability to diverse agroecosystems, and the practical challenges of field application underscore the need for a comprehensive understanding of the nuances involved. The success stories showcased in case studies offer valuable insights, but they also illuminate the gaps in our current understanding and point towards areas that demand further exploration. Environmental considerations take center stage as the narrative expands to encompass the broader ecological impact of microbial pest control strategies (Lengai et al., 2020). While the immediate goal is the targeted control of pest populations, the collateral effects on non-target organisms and the overall biodiversity of agricultural landscapes cannot be overlooked. The ecological footprint of microbial interventions becomes a critical consideration, shaping the discourse on the sustainability of these strategies. The potential for unintended consequences, such as the impact on beneficial insects or soil microbial communities, calls for a nuanced and cautious approach.

Regulatory frameworks emerge as a crucial aspect of the discourse, as the deployment of microbial pest control strategies necessitates a balance between innovation and risk mitigation. The absence of standardized protocols and guidelines for the registration and commercialization of microbial biopesticides poses challenges to their widespread adoption. Bridging the gap between scientific innovation and regulatory frameworks becomes imperative, ensuring that the deployment of beneficial microbes aligns with safety considerations and environmental stewardship (Mohanty et al., 2021).

The narrative unfolds against the backdrop of a changing climate and an evolving agricultural landscape. As we grapple with the challenges posed by climate change, the role of beneficial microbes becomes even more pronounced. The adaptability of these microbial allies to changing climatic conditions, their potential in mitigating the impact of climate stress on plants, and their contribution to resilient agroecosystems become integral components of the broader discourse on climate-smart agriculture. Looking towards the future, the story of beneficial microbes in agriculture remains dynamic and open-ended. The advent of advanced technologies, from CRISPR-based strategies to precision agriculture, adds new dimensions to the potential applications of microbial pest control (Seenivasagan and Babalola, 2021). The exploration of novel microbial strains, the fine-tuning of microbial formulations, and the integration of microbial approaches with emerging technologies represent avenues for ongoing research and innovation.

6.2 BENEFICIAL MICROBES IN AGRICULTURE

In the intricate tapestry of agriculture, beneficial microbes stand as microscopic architects, shaping the landscape of sustainable and resilient farming practices. These microbes, including bacteria, fungi, and viruses, have transcended their historical status as mere curiosities to emerge as pivotal players in the ongoing quest for ecologically conscious and economically viable agricultural systems.

6.2.1 *DIVERSITY OF BENEFICIAL MICROBES*

The microbial realm is teeming with diversity, each microorganism possessing unique attributes that can be harnessed for the betterment of agriculture. Bacteria, such as *Bacillus thuringiensis* (*Bt*), have long been recognized for their insecticidal properties. Fungi, exemplified by *Beauveria bassiana,* wield pathogenic prowess against a spectrum of insects. Viruses, particularly baculoviruses, stand out as highly specific bioinsecticides. This diversity allows for a tailored and nuanced approach to pest management, where specific microbes target specific pests, minimizing collateral damage to non-target organisms (Mącik et al., 2022).

6.2.2 *HISTORICAL ROOTS AND MODERN RESURGENCE*

The utilization of beneficial microbes is not a newfound revelation but a resurgence of ancient agricultural wisdom. Before the era of synthetic pesticides, farmers relied on the natural predilections of these microscopic allies to control pest populations. The modern resurgence of microbial strategies is a convergence of traditional knowledge with contemporary scientific understanding. It reflects a realization that the intricate dance between microbes, plants, and insects, honed over millennia, holds the key to sustainable and regenerative agriculture (Finkel et al., 2017).

6.2.3 *MODES OF ACTION*

The modes of action employed by beneficial microbes are both direct and indirect. In direct interactions, microorganisms act as pathogens or parasites, actively engaging with the physiology and life cycle of insect pests.

Indirect interactions involve a more subtle orchestration, where microbes influence plant physiology, inducing systemic resistance and arming plants with innate capabilities to fend off insect invasions (Yu et al., 2019). This dual strategy addresses not only the immediate pest challenge but also fortifies plants for future encounters.

6.2.4 CASE STUDIES AND PRACTICAL APPLICATIONS

The practicality of microbial pest control is underscored by an array of case studies demonstrating successful applications in the field. Microbial biopesticides, including various strains of *Bt* and entomopathogenic fungi (EPF), have found niches in organic farming and IPM programs (Porter et al., 2020). These success stories showcase the adaptability of microbial strategies to real-world agricultural settings and provide tangible evidence of their efficacy in curbing pest populations.

6.2.5 CHALLENGES AND CONSIDERATIONS

However, the path to widespread adoption of beneficial microbes is not without challenges. Scalability, adaptability to diverse agroecosystems, and the practical challenges of field application require careful consideration. Safety, both for humans and non-target organisms, is a paramount concern. The environmental footprint of microbial interventions and the potential for unintended consequences demand a nuanced and cautious approach. Bridging the gap between scientific innovation and regulatory frameworks is imperative to ensure the responsible deployment of microbial pest control strategies (Mahnert et al., 2018).

6.2.6 INTEGRATION INTO INTEGRATED PEST MANAGEMENT (IPM)

The integration of beneficial microbes into broader pest management strategies is a cornerstone of their application. IPM approaches, which combine multiple strategies for effective pest control, find a natural ally in beneficial microbes. The synergies between microbial strategies and other control methods, such as cultural practices and the judicious use of synthetic pesticides, represent a holistic approach to pest management (Deguine et al., 2021). It is a departure from singular reliance on chemical interventions, marking a transition towards a more integrated and sustainable agricultural paradigm.

6.2.7 ENVIRONMENTAL CONSIDERATIONS

The ecological impact of microbial pest control strategies extends beyond immediate pest control. Environmental considerations become integral to the discourse, with a focus on the impact on non-target organisms and the overall biodiversity of agricultural landscapes. The potential for unintended consequences, such as the impact on beneficial insects or soil microbial communities, calls for a careful balance between innovation and risk mitigation. Regulatory frameworks become crucial in ensuring that the deployment of beneficial microbes aligns with safety considerations and environmental stewardship (Karlsson et al., 2020).

6.2.8 CLIMATE-SMART AGRICULTURE

In the face of climate change, the adaptability of beneficial microbes becomes even more pronounced. These microbial allies contribute to resilient agroecosystems, mitigating the impact of climate stress on plants and insects alike. The narrative of climate-smart agriculture weaves into the broader story of beneficial microbes, positioning them as integral components in the quest for sustainable and climate-resilient farming practices (Azadi et al., 2021).

6.3 MODES OF ACTION OF BENEFICIAL MICROBES

The modes of action of beneficial microbes in agriculture are diverse and multifaceted, reflecting the intricate strategies employed by these microorganisms to contribute to pest management, plant health, and overall agroecosystem resilience. These modes of action can be broadly categorized into direct and indirect mechanisms, each playing a crucial role in the symbiotic relationships between microbes, plants, and pests (Köhl et al., 2019) (Figure 6.1).

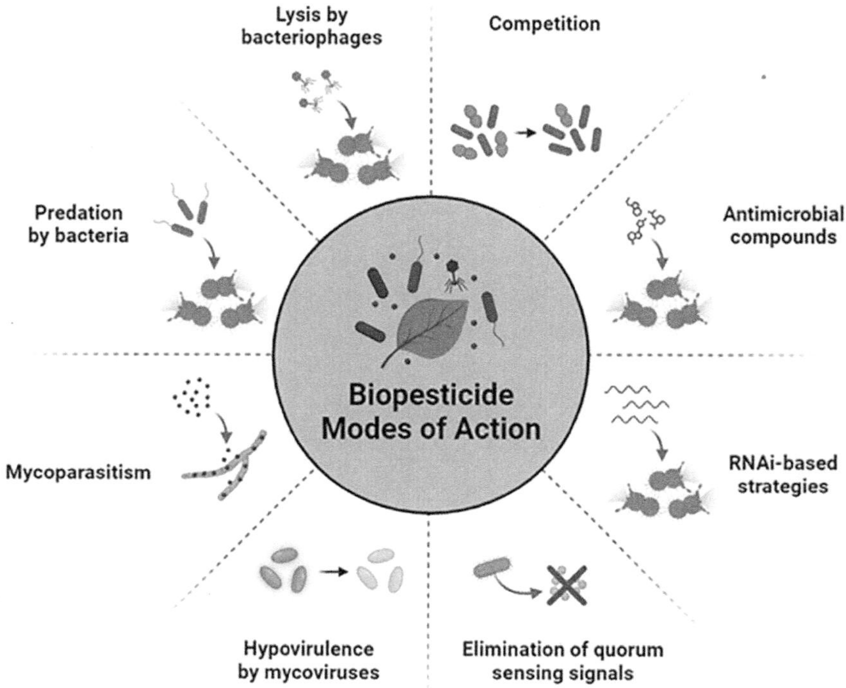

FIGURE 6.1 Mechanism of action of biochemical pesticides.

6.3.1 DIRECT MODES OF ACTION

6.3.1.1 PATHOGENICITY

- **Bacterial Pathogens (e.g., *Bacillus thuringiensis [Bt]*):** Certain bacteria produce toxins that are lethal to specific groups of insects. Upon ingestion, these toxins disrupt the insect's digestive system, leading to its demise. *Bt*, for instance, produces crystal proteins toxic to various insect larvae, making it a widely used bioinsecticide.
- **Fungal Pathogens (e.g., *Beauveria bassiana, Metarhizium anisopliae*):** EPF directly infect insects by attaching to their cuticle, penetrating the exoskeleton, and subsequently colonizing the insect host. These fungi are effective against a broad spectrum of insect pests.

- **Viral Pathogens (e.g., *Baculoviruses*):** Baculoviruses are specific to certain insect species. They infect the insect host, replicate within its cells, and ultimately lead to the death of the host. Baculoviruses are known for their host specificity, posing minimal risk to non-target organisms (James et al., 2021).

6.3.1.2 PARASITISM

- **Parasitic Wasps (e.g., *Trichogramma* spp.):** These tiny wasps lay their eggs inside the eggs of insect pests, preventing the development of the pest larvae. The emerging wasp larvae consume the pest eggs, providing a natural and targeted form of biological control (Berg et al., 2021).

6.3.2 INDIRECT MODES OF ACTION

6.3.2.1 INDUCED SYSTEMIC RESISTANCE (ISR)

- **Bacterial Induction (e.g., *Pseudomonas* spp.):** Beneficial bacteria can induce systemic resistance in plants. When these bacteria colonize the plant's rhizosphere, they trigger a cascade of biochemical responses within the plant, enhancing its ability to defend against a broad spectrum of pests and pathogens. This systemic resistance is a form of long-lasting immunization for the plant (Hesham et al., 2021).

6.3.2.2 PLANT-MEDIATED INTERACTIONS

- **Volatile Compound Emission:** Beneficial microbes influence the emission of volatile organic compounds (VOCs) by plants. These compounds serve as signaling molecules that can attract natural enemies of pests or repel the pests themselves. The intricate communication network between plants, microbes, and insects plays a crucial role in shaping the overall ecology of the agroecosystem (O'Callaghan et al., 2022).
- **Root Exudates:** Microbes in the rhizosphere influence the composition of root exudates, chemical compounds released by

plant roots. These exudates can attract or repel specific organisms in the soil, influencing the plant's interactions with both beneficial and harmful soil-dwelling organisms (Wang et al., 2020).

6.3.2.3 NUTRIENT COMPETITION AND EXCLUSION

- **Rhizosphere Competition (e.g., Mycorrhizal Fungi):** Beneficial microbes in the rhizosphere, such as mycorrhizal fungi, form symbiotic relationships with plants, enhancing nutrient uptake. By doing so, they outcompete potential pathogens for essential nutrients, indirectly contributing to plant health and resilience (Posta and Duc, 2020).

6.3.2.4 PRODUCTION OF ANTAGONISTIC COMPOUNDS

- **Antibiotic Production (e.g., *Streptomyces* spp.):** Some beneficial bacteria produce antibiotics that suppress the growth of pathogenic microorganisms. This can help in controlling soil-borne diseases and enhancing the overall health of the agroecosystem (Ramakuwela et al., 2020).
- **Antifungal Metabolites (e.g., *Trichoderma* spp.):** Certain fungi, like *Trichoderma*, produce antifungal metabolites that inhibit the growth of pathogenic fungi. This antagonistic activity contributes to disease suppression and promotes plant health (Bamisile et al., 2019).

6.3.3 DUAL MODES OF ACTION

6.3.3.1 DUAL ROLES IN PEST MANAGEMENT AND NUTRIENT CYCLING

- **Entomopathogenic Nematodes:** These microscopic worms not only infect and kill insect pests directly but also contribute to nutrient cycling. As they parasitize insects, they release nutrients into the soil upon completing their life cycle, benefitting plants and enhancing soil fertility (Gouda et al., 2018).

6.3.3.2 *SYMBIOTIC RELATIONSHIPS*

- **Mycorrhizal Associations:** Mycorrhizal fungi form symbiotic relationships with plant roots, aiding in nutrient absorption. Simultaneously, they can indirectly influence pest populations by enhancing plant health and vigor, making plants more resilient to pest attacks.

6.4 BENEFICIAL MICROBES AND INSECT PEST MANAGEMENT

In the intricate tapestry of agriculture, the symbiotic relationship between beneficial microbes and insect pest management emerges as a dynamic and ecologically conscious approach. This alliance harnesses the intrinsic capabilities of various microorganisms, including bacteria, fungi, and viruses, to curtail the impact of insect pests on crops. The intricate dance between these beneficial microbes and their insect counterparts unfolds as a multifaceted strategy within the broader framework of IPM (Timmusk et al., 2018).

6.4.1 *DIVERSITY AND FUNCTIONS OF BENEFICIAL MICROBES*

Beneficial microbes constitute a diverse array of microorganisms, each wielding unique tools in the battle against insect pests. Bacteria, exemplified by *Bacillus thuringiensis* (*Bt*), produce toxins lethal to specific insect groups. Fungi, notably *Beauveria bassiana* and *Metarhizium anisopliae*, are entomopathogenic, infecting and debilitating a wide range of insects. Viruses, such as baculoviruses, are highly specific to certain insect species, making them potent candidates for bioinsecticides (Wang et al., 2021).

6.4.2 *DIRECT MECHANISMS OF ACTION*

Beneficial microbes exert their influence through both direct and indirect mechanisms. In direct interactions, these microorganisms act as pathogens or parasites, actively engaging with the physiology and life cycle of the target insect pests (Subrahmanyam et al., 2020). For instance, *Bt* bacteria produce proteins toxic to specific insects upon ingestion, leading to their demise. EPF, on the other hand, adhere to the insect cuticle, penetrate the exoskeleton, and subsequently colonize the insect host.

6.4.3 *INDIRECT MECHANISMS AND PLANT-MICROBE-INSECT INTERACTIONS*

The influence of beneficial microbes extends beyond direct confrontation with insect pests. Indirect mechanisms involve the intricate interplay between microbes, plants, and insects. Microbes induce systemic resistance in plants, priming them to respond more effectively to insect attacks. This phenomenon, known as induced systemic resistance (ISR), marks a departure from pest control methods by empowering plants to actively participate in their own defense (Bertola et al., 2021). Moreover, beneficial microbes contribute to the modulation of plant volatiles, adding a layer of complexity to plant-microbe-insect interactions. The emission of VOCs by plants serves as a form of communication, influencing the behavior of both insects and their natural enemies. Beneficial microbes play a role in shaping this aromatic dialogue, either deterring insect pests or attracting predators and parasitoids that serve as allies in pest management (Subrahmanyam et al., 2020) (Figure 6.2).

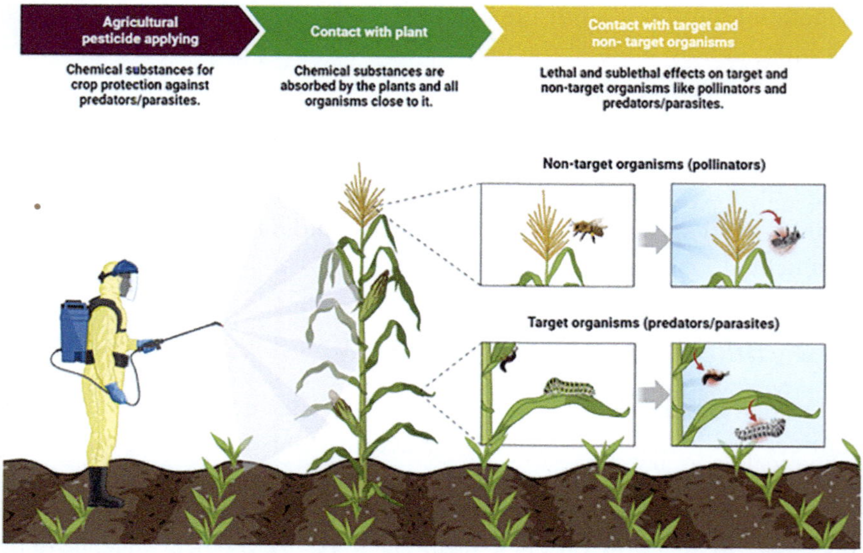

FIGURE 6.2 Utilizing plant growth-promoting rhizobacteria (PGPR) as biofertilizers and biopesticides.

6.5 BACTERIAL INSECTICIDES: HARNESSING THE POWER OF BENEFICIAL BACTERIA FOR PEST CONTROL

Bacterial insecticides have emerged as pivotal components in sustainable pest management within agriculture. These insecticides, primarily utilizing the bacterium *Bacillus thuringiensis* (*Bt*), present a targeted and environmentally friendly approach to controlling specific pest populations. The mechanisms of action of bacterial insecticides revolve around the production of toxins, notably *Bt* toxins, during the sporulation phase of the bacteria's life cycle (de Bruijn et al., 2022). These toxins, specific to certain insect groups, disrupt the digestive systems of target pests, leading to their paralysis and eventual demise. The high specificity and selectivity of these toxins minimize harm to non-target organisms, setting bacterial insecticides apart from broad-spectrum chemical alternatives.

The advantages of bacterial insecticides extend beyond their environmental friendliness. They contribute to resistance management, with a lower likelihood of pests developing resistance compared to chemical pesticides. Compatibility with IPM approaches allows for their seamless integration into holistic pest control strategies. Additionally, bacterial insecticides exhibit reduced environmental impact due to their rapid breakdown, aligning with principles of sustainable agriculture (Goh et al., 2023).

However, challenges and considerations exist. Bacterial insecticides may have a limited spectrum of control, requiring alternative strategies for non-susceptible pests. Their efficacy can be influenced by environmental conditions, necessitating optimal circumstances for maximum effectiveness. Practical challenges in application, including formulation and coverage considerations, are also areas of ongoing research. Bacterial insecticides find applications in various crops, including cotton, corn, vegetables, and fruits, effectively targeting caterpillar pests. They are also employed in forestry to control defoliating insects and in mosquito control, with *Bt israelensis* targeting mosquito larvae in standing water. Looking ahead, biotechnological advancements—such as the development of genetically modified crops expressing *Bt* toxins—represent a promising avenue. Efforts are underway to broaden the spectrum of bacterial insecticides to target additional pest species by exploring new bacterial strains with diverse toxin profiles (Qasim, 2023) (Figure 6.3).

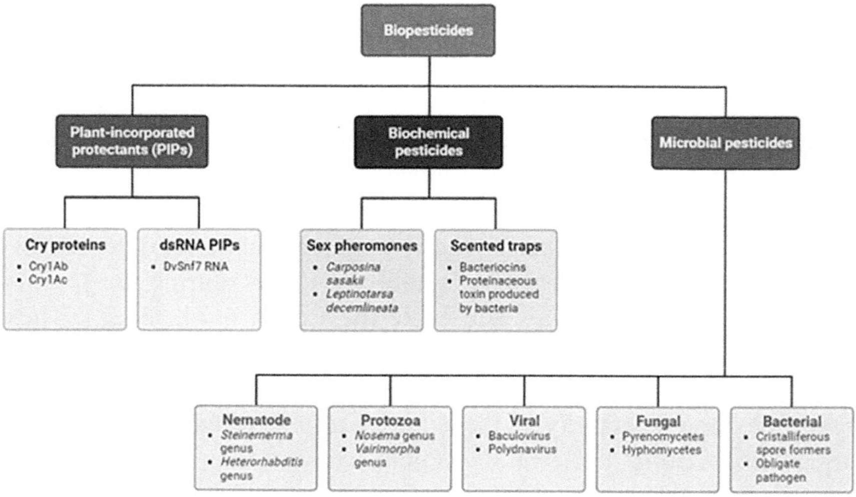

FIGURE 6.3 Categorization of biopesticides.

6.6 FUNGAL INSECTICIDES

Fungal insecticides have emerged as influential tools in sustainable pest management, leveraging the capabilities of EPF to control specific insect pests. Unlike chemical alternatives, these insecticides present a targeted and environmentally conscious approach to pest control. The primary mechanism of action involves EPF, such as *Beauveria bassiana* and *Metarhizium anisopliae*, infecting and colonizing insect hosts (Miller et al., 2019). These fungi adhere to the insect cuticle, penetrate the exoskeleton, and subsequently proliferate within the host, leading to its demise. The specificity of these fungi to certain insect species minimizes harm to non-target organisms, making fungal insecticides a valuable component in IPM strategies. Advantages of fungal insecticides include their environmental friendliness (Ahmad, 2020). They pose minimal risk to beneficial insects, birds, and mammals, contributing to the preservation of ecological balance. Their mode of action is multifaceted, reducing the likelihood of pests developing resistance compared to chemical pesticides. Moreover, the rapid breakdown of fungal insecticides minimizes their environmental persistence, aligning with principles of sustainable agriculture. Despite their advantages, fungal insecticides face challenges. Practical considerations such as formulation, application methods, and environmental conditions can impact their efficacy. Innovations in application technologies are ongoing to address scalability and practicality issues. Applications of fungal insecticides span various crops, including cotton, vegetables, and fruits, effectively controlling a range of insect pests (Bamisile et al., 2021). Their efficacy extends to soil-dwelling pests, making them valuable in IPM programs. Looking forward, ongoing research explores biotechnological advancements and the development of novel fungal strains. These endeavors aim to enhance the effectiveness and broaden the spectrum of fungal insecticides, making them more versatile in addressing diverse pest challenges.

6.7 VIRAL INSECTICIDES

Viral insecticides represent a promising and environmentally friendly approach to pest management in agriculture. These insecticides harness the natural pathogenicity of viruses, specifically baculoviruses, to control specific insect pests. Unlike chemical pesticides, viral insecticides offer targeted and selective control while minimizing harm to non-target organisms and ecosystems. The primary mechanism of action involves baculoviruses infecting the target insect host. Baculoviruses, such as nucleopolyhedroviruses (NPVs) and granuloviruses (GVs), are highly specific to certain insect species (Huang et al., 2020). The viruses typically enter the insect through ingestion, inhalation, or contact with the cuticle. Once inside the insect, the virus replicates, causing a systemic infection that ultimately leads to the death of the host. The virus then produces occlusion bodies (OBs), which are protein crystals containing the viral particles, facilitating the infection of other susceptible insects (Ahirwar et al., 2020).

The advantages of viral insecticides are evident in their high specificity and selectivity. They are effective against specific insect pests while posing minimal risk to beneficial organisms, such as pollinators and natural enemies of pests. Additionally, the risk of target pests developing resistance to viral insecticides is relatively low compared to chemical pesticides. Viral insecticides contribute to IPM strategies, aligning with principles of sustainable agriculture (Shukla et al., 2019). Their environmentally friendly nature, low toxicity to non-target organisms, and reduced impact on ecosystems make them valuable tools in fostering balanced and resilient agroecosystems. Despite their advantages, challenges exist in the commercialization and practical application of viral insecticides.

Issues such as stability, formulation, and the need for improved delivery methods are areas of ongoing research. Advances in biotechnological approaches and formulation technologies aim to address these challenges, enhancing the efficacy and feasibility of viral insecticides in the field. Applications of viral insecticides extend across various crops, including fruits, vegetables, and row crops. They are particularly effective against lepidopteran pests, such as caterpillars, and have shown promise in forestry and urban pest management (Jing et al., 2021).

As research continues, the development of novel viral strains and the exploration of synergies with other pest management strategies hold promise for expanding the use of viral insecticides. The ongoing evolution of these insecticides reflects a commitment to sustainable and ecologically conscious pest control practices in agriculture.

6.8 BENEFICIAL MICROBES AND PLANT-MICROBE-INSECT INTERACTIONS: A TRIPARTITE SYMPHONY

In the intricate dance of agricultural ecosystems, beneficial microbes play a pivotal role in shaping the interactions between plants and insects. This tripartite interplay forms a dynamic web of relationships that influences plant health, pest resistance, and overall agroecosystem resilience (Zytynska, 2021). This overview explores the multifaceted interactions between beneficial microbes, plants, and insects, highlighting the mechanisms through which microbes contribute to sustainable and IPM strategies. Beneficial microbes encompass a diverse array of bacteria, fungi, viruses, and nematodes that form symbiotic relationships with plants. This intricate network extends to interactions with insect herbivores, shaping the ecological dynamics within agricultural systems.

6.8.1 DIRECT INTERACTIONS

1. **Microbial-Induced Resistance (MIR):** Beneficial microbes can induce resistance in plants against insect herbivores. This phenomenon, known as MIR, involves the activation of plant defense mechanisms in response to microbial colonization. The primed plants exhibit enhanced resistance to insect pests (Rastegari et al., 2020).

2. **Microbial Volatile Organic Compounds (mVOCs):** Beneficial microbes release VOCs that serve as chemical signals. These mVOCs play a role in attracting or repelling insects. For example, certain microbes can emit compounds that attract the natural enemies of insect pests, contributing to biological control (Mącik et al., 2022).

6.8.2 INDIRECT INTERACTIONS

1. **Nutrient Cycling and Plant Health:** Beneficial microbes enhance nutrient cycling in the rhizosphere, promoting plant health. Healthy plants are more resilient to pest attacks, and the competition for nutrients between beneficial microbes and pathogens indirectly contributes to disease suppression.
2. **Induced Systemic Resistance (ISR):** Certain bacteria, such as Pseudomonas spp., induce systemic resistance in plants. This systemic response primes the entire plant for enhanced defense against a spectrum of pests, providing a long-lasting and broad-spectrum form of protection.

6.8.3 MICROBES AS INSECT PEST ANTAGONISTS

1. **Entomopathogenic Fungi:** Fungi like *Beauveria bassiana* and *Metarhizium anisopliae* are entomopathogenic, infecting and killing insect pests. These fungi can form associations with plant roots, offering a dual benefit by enhancing plant health and providing a natural form of pest control (Bertola et al., 2021).
2. **Bacterial Insecticides (e.g., *Bacillus thuringiensis* [*Bt*]):** *Bt* bacteria produce insecticidal toxins that specifically target certain insect pests. When applied as bioinsecticides, *Bt* contributes to pest control without harming non-target organisms, showcasing the targeted impact of beneficial microbes.

6.8.4 SYMBIOTIC RELATIONSHIPS

1. **Mycorrhizal Associations:** Mycorrhizal fungi form symbiotic relationships with plant roots, aiding in nutrient absorption. The enhanced nutrient uptake indirectly influences pest populations by

promoting plant health and vigor, making them more resilient to pest attacks.

2. **Rhizobacteria and Root Exudates:** Rhizobacteria influence the composition of root exudates, chemical compounds released by plant roots. These exudates can attract or repel specific organisms in the soil, shaping the plant's interactions with both beneficial and harmful soil-dwelling insects.

6.8.5 INTEGRATION INTO PEST MANAGEMENT

1. **Biological Control:** Beneficial microbes are integral to biological control strategies. The release of natural enemies, attracted by microbial signals, can provide effective and sustainable pest management.
2. **Microbial Inoculants:** The application of microbial inoculants, such as biopesticides containing beneficial microbes, has become a key component of IPM programs. These inoculants contribute to pest control while promoting overall agroecosystem health.

6.9 INTEGRATION OF BENEFICIAL MICROBES IN INTEGRATED PEST MANAGEMENT (IPM): A HOLISTIC APPROACH TO SUSTAINABLE AGRICULTURE

IPM represents a comprehensive strategy for pest control that emphasizes ecological balance, minimal environmental impact, and sustainable agricultural practices. Within the framework of IPM, the integration of beneficial microbes plays a central role, offering targeted and environmentally friendly solutions to pest challenges (Naik et al., 2019). This overview explores the key components of incorporating beneficial microbes into IPM programs, highlighting their diverse roles in promoting plant health, enhancing pest resistance, and contributing to overall agroecosystem sustainability. IPM is a strategic and multifaceted approach to pest control that seeks to minimize the use of synthetic pesticides while promoting effective and sustainable solutions. IPM integrates a range of practices, including biological control, cultural practices, mechanical methods, and the judicious use of chemical pesticides when necessary (Porter et al., 2020).

6.9.1 ROLE OF BENEFICIAL MICROBES IN IPM

1. **Biological Control:** Beneficial microbes, including bacteria, fungi, viruses, and nematodes, act as natural enemies of pests. They contribute to biological control by directly suppressing pest populations or by influencing the behavior and ecology of pests.
2. **Microbial Induced Resistance (MIR):** Beneficial microbes induce resistance in plants against pest attacks. This MIR primes plants to mount a more effective defense against a range of pests, reducing the need for chemical interventions.
3. **Enhanced Nutrient Uptake:** Mycorrhizal fungi form symbiotic associations with plant roots, enhancing nutrient uptake. This improved nutrient status makes plants more resilient to pest attacks, contributing to a healthier and more robust agroecosystem.

6.9.2 COMPONENTS OF MICROBIAL INTEGRATION IN IPM

1. **Microbial Inoculants:** Application of microbial inoculants, such as biopesticides containing beneficial microbes, is a key component of IPM. These inoculants provide targeted pest control without negatively impacting non-target organisms.
2. **Crop Rotation and Microbial Communities:** Crop rotation practices influence the composition of soil microbial communities. The diversity and health of these communities contribute to pest suppression and overall soil fertility, aligning with IPM principles.
3. **Conservation of Natural Enemies:** Beneficial microbes contribute to the conservation of natural enemies of pests. By enhancing the habitat and resources available to predators and parasitoids, microbes indirectly support biological control within the agroecosystem.

6.9.3 ADVANTAGES OF MICROBIAL INTEGRATION

1. **Environmentally Friendly:** The targeted nature of microbial interventions minimizes environmental impact. Beneficial microbes pose little risk to non-target organisms, preserving

biodiversity and reducing the ecological footprint associated with chemical pesticides.

2. **Resistance Management:** The risk of pests developing resistance to microbial interventions is generally lower compared to synthetic pesticides. This aligns with IPM principles, promoting long-term and sustainable pest control (Ahirwar et al., 2020).
3. **Soil Health and Fertility:** Beneficial microbes contribute to soil health and fertility. By enhancing nutrient cycling, improving soil structure, and suppressing soil-borne pathogens, these microbes create a foundation for sustainable crop production (Qadri et al., 2020).

6.10 CONCLUSION AND FUTURE PROSPECTS

The utilization of beneficial microbes for insect management has marked a transformative shift in agricultural practices, offering sustainable solutions for pest control and ecosystem balance. The journey so far has uncovered a myriad of advantages, showcasing the potential of these microbes to revolutionize pest management strategies. The direct actions of EPF and bacteria, coupled with the induction of systemic resistance in plants, exemplify the sophistication and sustainability of microbial approaches. Mycorrhizal associations, microbial volatile organic compounds (mVOCs), and the orchestration of natural enemies highlight the complexity of the microbial toolkit, guiding agriculture away from reliance on chemical pesticides and towards greater environmental harmony.

The environmentally friendly nature of microbial interventions has become a cornerstone of their success, mitigating adverse effects on non-target organisms and preserving biodiversity. The lower risk of resistance development, in comparison to synthetic pesticides, underscores the long-term efficacy and resilience of microbial strategies. Additionally, the positive influence of beneficial microbes on soil health and fertility underscores the interconnectedness of healthy soils, robust plants, and effective pest management. Looking to the future, promising prospects lie in biotechnological advancements, the development of microbial consortia, precision agriculture, and a deeper understanding of microbial interactions. These avenues of exploration hold the potential to further optimize the integration of beneficial microbes into agricultural practices, enhancing their effectiveness while minimizing environmental impact. As agriculture navigates the evolving landscape of sustainability, beneficial microbes stand as key allies, guiding the path towards a more resilient, balanced, and ecologically conscious agricultural future. The role of these microbes is not merely a component of sustainable agriculture; it is a transformative narrative, reshaping the story of agriculture towards enduring sustainability, balance, and environmental stewardship.

KEYWORDS

- **beneficial microbes**
- **biodiversity**
- **crop rotation**
- **microbial consortia**
- **microbial-induced resistance**
- **microbial volatile organic compounds**
- **soil health**

REFERENCES

Ahirwar, N. K., Singh, R., Chaurasia, S., Chandra, R., & Ramana, S. (2020). Effective role of beneficial microbes in achieving the sustainable agriculture and eco-friendly environment development goals: A review. *Frontiers in Microbiology*, *5*, 111–123.

Ahmad, K. S. (2020). Remedial potential of bacterial and fungal strains (*Bacillus subtilis*, *Aspergillus niger*, *Aspergillus flavus* and *Penicillium chrysogenum*) against organochlorine insecticide Endosulfan. *Folia Microbiological*, *65*(5), 801–810.

Azadi, H., Moghaddam, S. M., Burkart, S., Mahmoudi, H., Van Passel, S., Kurban, A., & Lopez-Carr, D. (2021). Rethinking resilient agriculture: From climate-smart agriculture to vulnerable-smart agriculture. *Journal of Cleaner Production*, *319*, 128602.

Bamisile, B. S., Akutse, K. S., Siddiqui, J. A., & Xu, Y. (2021). Model application of entomopathogenic fungi as alternatives to chemical pesticides: Prospects, challenges, and insights for next-generation sustainable agriculture. *Frontiers in Plant Science*, *12*, 741804.

Bamisile, B. S., Dash, C. K., Akutse, K. S., Qasim, M., Ramos Aguila, L. C., Wang, F., et al. (2019). Endophytic *Beauveria bassiana* in foliar-treated *Citrus limon* plants acting as a growth suppressor to three successive generations of *Diaphorina citri* Kuwayama (Hemiptera: Liviidae). *Insects*, *10*, 176.

Berg, G., Kusstatscher, P., Abdelfattah, A., Cernava, T., & Smalla, K. (2021). Microbiome modulation—Toward a better understanding of plant microbiome response to microbial inoculants. *Frontiers in Microbiology, 12*, 650610.

Bertola, M., Ferrarini, A., & Visioli, G. (2021). Improvement of soil microbial diversity through sustainable agricultural practices and its evaluation by -omics approaches: A perspective for the environment, food quality and human safety. *Microorganisms, 9*(7), 1400.

de Bruijn, F. J., Smidt, H., Cocolin, L. S., Sauer, M., Dowling, D. N., & Thomashow, L. (2022). *Good Microbes in Medicine, Food Production, Biotechnology, Bioremediation, and Agriculture*. John Wiley & Sons.

Deguine, J. P., Aubertot, J. N., Flor, R. J., Lescourret, F., Wyckhuys, K. A., & Ratnadass, A. (2021). Integrated pest management: Good intentions, hard realities. A review. *Agronomy for Sustainable Development, 41*(3), 38.

Elnahal, A. S., El-Saadony, M. T., Saad, A. M., Desoky, E. S. M., El-Tahan, A. M., Rady, M. M., & El-Tarabily, K. A. (2022). The use of microbial inoculants for biological control, plant growth promotion, and sustainable agriculture: A review. *European Journal of Plant Pathology, 162*(4), 759–792.

Finkel, O. M., Castrillo, G., Paredes, S. H., González, I. S., & Dangl, J. L. (2017). Understanding and exploiting plant beneficial microbes. *Current Opinion in Plant Biology, 38*, 155–163.

Goh, Y. J., DeYoung, B. J., Dove, N. C., Johnson, B. R., Martz, M. K., Mel, M., & Videau, P. (2023). Harnessing the microbial world for human benefit. *Trends in Biotechnology*.

Gouda, S., Kerry, R. G., Das, G., Paramithiotis, S., Shin, H. S., & Patra, J. K. (2018). Revitalization of plant growth promoting rhizobacteria for sustainable development in agriculture. *Microbiological Research, 206*, 131–140.

Hesham, A. E. L., Kaur, T., Devi, R., Kour, D., Prasad, S., Yadav, N., & Yadav, A. N. (2021). Current trends in microbial biotechnology for agricultural sustainability: Conclusion and future challenges. In *Current Trends in Microbial Biotechnology for Sustainable Agriculture* (pp. 555–572).

Huang, X., Li, T., Shan, X., Lu, R., Hao, M., Lv, M., & Xu, H. (2020). High value-added use of citrus industrial wastes in agriculture: Semi synthesis and anti-tobacco mosaic virus/insecticidal activities of ester derivatives of limonin modified in the B ring. *Journal of Agricultural and Food Chemistry, 68*(44), 12241–12251.

James, G., Das, B. C., Jose, S., & VJ, R. K. (2021). *Bacillus* as an aquaculture friendly microbe. *Aquaculture International, 29*, 323–353.

Jing, W. A. N., Huang, C., Li, C. Y., Zhou, H. X., Ren, Y. L., Li, Z. Y., & Wan, F. H. (2021). Biology, invasion and management of the agricultural invader: Fall armyworm, *Spodoptera frugiperda* (Lepidoptera: Noctuidae). *Journal of Integrative Agriculture, 20*(3), 646–663.

Karlsson Green, K., Stenberg, J. A., & Lankinen, Å. (2020). Making sense of integrated pest management (IPM) in the light of evolution. *Evolutionary Applications, 13*(8), 1791–1805.

Köhl, J., Kolnaar, R., & Ravensberg, W. J. (2019). Mode of action of microbial biological control agents against plant diseases: Relevance beyond efficacy. *Frontiers in Plant Science, 845*.

Lengai, G. M., Muthomi, J. W., & Mbega, E. R. (2020). Phytochemical activity and role of botanical pesticides in pest management for sustainable agricultural crop production. *Scientific African*, *7*, e00239.

Mącik, M., Gryta, A., Sas-Paszt, L., & Frąc, M. (2022). Composition, activity and diversity of bacterial and fungal communities' responses to inputs of phosphorus fertilizer enriched with beneficial microbes in degraded *Brunic Arenosol. Land Degradation & Development*, *33*(6), 844–865.

Mahnert, A., Haratani, M., Schmuck, M., & Berg, G. (2018). Enriching beneficial microbial diversity of indoor plants and their surrounding built environment with bio stimulants. *Frontiers in Microbiology*, *9*, 2985.

Miller, L. K., Lingg, A. J., & Bulla, L. A. (2019). Bacterial, viral, and fungal insecticides. In *Biotechnology and Biological Frontiers* (pp. 214–229). Routledge.

Mohanty, P., Singh, P. K., Chakraborty, D., Mishra, S., & Pattnaik, R. (2021). Insight into the role of PGPR in sustainable agriculture and environment. *Frontiers in Sustainable Food Systems*, *5*, 667150.

Naik, K., Mishra, S., Srichandan, H., Singh, P. K., & Sarangi, P. K. (2019). Plant growth promoting microbes: Potential link to sustainable agriculture and environment. *Biocatalysis and Agricultural Biotechnology*, *21*, 101326.

O'Callaghan, M., Ballard, R. A., & Wright, D. (2022). Soil microbial inoculants for sustainable agriculture: Limitations and opportunities. *Soil Use and Management*, *38*(3), 1340–1369.

Olaniyan, O. T., & Adetunji, C. O. (2021). Biochemical role of beneficial microorganisms: An overview on recent development in environmental and agro science. In *Microbial Rejuvenation of Polluted Environment: Volume 3* (pp. 21–33).

Ortiz, A., & Sansinenea, E. (2022). The role of beneficial microorganisms in soil quality and plant health. *Sustainability*, *14*(9), 5358.

Porter, S. S., Bantay, R., Friel, C. A., Garoutte, A., Gdanetz, K., Ibarreta, K., & Friesen, M. L. (2020). Beneficial microbes ameliorate abiotic and biotic sources of stress on plants. *Functional Ecology*, *34*(10), 2075–2086.

Posta, K., & Duc, N. H. (2020). Benefits of arbuscular mycorrhizal fungi application to crop production under water scarcity. In *Drought Detection and Solutions*.

Qadri, M., Short, S., Gast, K., Hernandez, J., & Wong, A. C. N. (2020). Microbiome innovation in agriculture: Development of microbial-based tools for insect pest management. *Frontiers in Sustainable Food Systems*, *4*, 547751.

Qasim, M. (2023). Beneficial microbes in plant health: From biocontrol agent to plant growth promoting rhizobacteria. *International Journal of Research and Advances in Agricultural Sciences*, *2*(3), 39–49.

Rai, P. K., Singh, M., Anand, K., Saurabh, S., Kaur, T., Kour, D., & Kumar, M. (2020). Role and potential applications of plant growth-promoting rhizobacteria for sustainable agriculture. In *New and Future Developments in Microbial Biotechnology and Bioengineering* (pp. 49–60). Elsevier.

Ramakuwela, T., Hatting, J., Bock, C., Vega, F. E., Wells, L., Mbata, G. N., & Shapiro-Ilan, D. (2020). Establishment of *Beauveria bassiana* as a fungal endophyte in pecan (*Carya illinoinensis*) seedlings and its virulence against pecan insect pests. *Biological Control*, *140*, 104102.

Rastegari, A. A., Yadav, A. N., & Yadav, N. (2020). *New and Future Developments in Microbial Biotechnology and Bioengineering: Trends of Microbial Biotechnology for Sustainable Agriculture and Biomedicine Systems: Diversity and Functional Perspectives*. Elsevier.

Ray, P., Lakshmanan, V., Labbé, J. L., & Craven, K. D. (2020). Microbe to microbiome: A paradigm shift in the application of microorganisms for sustainable agriculture. *Frontiers in Microbiology*, *11*, 622926.

Ruiu, L. (2020). Plant-growth-promoting bacteria (PGPB) against insects and other agricultural pests. *Agronomy*, *10*(6), 861.

Seenivasagan, R., & Babalola, O. O. (2021). Utilization of microbial consortia as biofertilizers and biopesticides for the production of feasible agricultural product. *Biology*, *10*(11), 1111.

Shukla, N., Singh, E. A. N. A., Kabadwa, B. C., Sharma, R., & Kumar, J. (2019). Present status and future prospects of bio-agents in agriculture. *International Journal of Current Microbiology and Applied Sciences*, *8*(4), 2138–2153.

Subrahmanyam, G., Kumar, A., Sandilya, S. P., Chutia, M., & Yadav, A. N. (2020). Diversity, plant growth promoting attributes, and agricultural applications of rhizosphere microbes. In *Plant Microbiomes for Sustainable Agriculture* (pp. 1–52).

Thakur, N., Kaur, S., Tomar, P., Thakur, S., & Yadav, A. N. (2020). Microbial biopesticides: Current status and advancement for sustainable agriculture and environment. In *New and Future Developments in Microbial Biotechnology and Bioengineering* (pp. 243–282). Elsevier.

Timmusk, S., Seisenbaeva, G., & Behers, L. (2018). Titania (TiO_2) nanoparticles enhance the performance of growth-promoting rhizobacteria. *Scientific Reports*, *8*, 617.

Trivedi, P., Mattupalli, C., Eversole, K., & Leach, J. E. (2021). Enabling sustainable agriculture through understanding and enhancement of microbiomes. *New Phytologist*, *230*(6), 2129–2147.

Wang, F., Adams, C. A., Yang, W., Sun, Y., & Shi, Z. (2020). Benefits of arbuscular mycorrhizal fungi in reducing organic contaminant residues in crops: Implications for cleaner agricultural production. *Critical Reviews in Environmental Science and Technology*, *50*(15), 1580–1612.

Wang, G., Bei, S., Li, J., Bao, X., Zhang, J., Schultz, P. A., & Zhang, J. (2021). Soil microbial legacy drives crop diversity advantage: Linking ecological plant–soil feedback with agricultural intercropping. *Journal of Applied Ecology*, *58*(3), 496–506.

Yu, K., Pieterse, C. M., Bakker, P. A., & Berendsen, R. L. (2019). Beneficial microbes going underground of root immunity. *Plant, Cell & Environment*, *42*(10), 2860–2870.

Zytynska, S. E. (2021). Embracing the complexity of plant–microbe–insect interactions under a changing climate for sustainable agriculture. *Current Opinion in Insect Science*, *44*, 89–94.

CHAPTER 7

Harnessing Soil Microorganisms for Sustainable Agriculture: Role of Biofortification Strategies

PRITI PAL,[1] AKHILESH KUMAR SINGH,[2]
PRAKASH KUMAR SARANGI,[3] UTTAM KUMAR SAHOO,[4]
ANAND PRAKASH,[2] and BRIJESH PANDEY[2,*]

[1]*Amity Institute of Biotechnology, Amity University Uttar Pradesh, Lucknow Campus, Lucknow, India*

[2]*Department of Biotechnology, School of Life Sciences, Mahatma Gandhi Central University, Motihari, Bihar, India*

[3]*College of Agriculture, Central Agricultural University, Imphal, Manipur, India*

[4]*Department of Forestry, Mizoram University, Aizawl, Mizoram, India*

*Corresponding authors

ABSTRACT

In the face of global challenges such as population growth, climate change, and nutrient depletion in agricultural soils, sustainable agricultural practices are imperative to ensure food security and nutrition. Biofortification, the process of enhancing the nutrient content of crops through natural means, has emerged as a promising strategy. This abstract explores the pivotal role of soil microorganisms in biofortification and their contribution to sustainable agriculture. Soil microorganisms, including bacteria, fungi, and archaea, play a fundamental role in nutrient cycling and availability in the rhizosphere. Their interactions with plant roots influence nutrient uptake,

Biotechnology for Sustainable Agriculture: Innovative Approaches and Strategies.
Prakash Kumar Sarangi (Ed)

DOI: 10.1201/9781779642998-7

enhance nutrient mobilization, and contribute to the synthesis of bioactive compounds. This paper reviews the diverse mechanisms employed by soil microorganisms, such as nitrogen-fixation, phosphate solubilization, and production of plant growth-promoting substances, to positively impact plant nutrition and health. Furthermore, the utilization of beneficial microbes as biofertilizers and biopesticides is discussed, emphasizing their potential to reduce the dependence on chemical inputs and mitigate environmental risks associated with conventional agricultural practices.

7.1 INTRODUCTION

As the global population continues to burgeon, exceeding nine billion by 2050 according to United Nations projections, ensuring food security and nutritional sufficiency presents an intricate challenge for the agricultural sector. Concurrently, the escalating impacts of climate change and the depletion of essential nutrients in agricultural soils further exacerbate this challenge. In response, sustainable agricultural practices are gaining prominence, seeking to harmonize increased food production with environmental conservation and long-term soil health (Dhiman et al., 2023).

At the heart of this pursuit lies the concept of biofortification, a transformative approach aimed at enhancing the nutritional quality of crops through natural processes. Biofortification stands as a beacon of hope in addressing widespread malnutrition, particularly in regions where access to diverse and nutrient-rich diets is limited. In this context, soil microorganisms emerge as unsung heroes, playing a pivotal role in orchestrating nutrient dynamics within the rhizosphere and influencing the overall health and productivity of crops (Roriz et al., 2020).

Understanding the intrinsic link between soil microorganisms and biofortification requires an exploration of the broader landscape of global agriculture. Traditional methods of addressing nutrient deficiencies have often involved the application of synthetic fertilizers, contributing to environmental pollution, soil degradation, and unsustainable farming practices. In contrast, biofortification harnesses the natural symbiosis between plants and soil microorganisms to fortify crops with essential nutrients (Jaiswal et al., 2022). This marks a paradigm shift towards a more sustainable and environmentally conscious approach to agricultural development. The intricate dance between soil microorganisms and plant roots unfolds in the rhizosphere, a dynamic interface where nutrient exchanges and microbial interactions shape the health and resilience of crops. Nitrogen-fixing bacteria, phosphate-solubilizing fungi, and a myriad of other microorganisms engage in a complex symphony of biochemical processes that contribute to nutrient cycling and availability (Daly et al., 2017). This chapter delves into the multifaceted mechanisms through which soil microorganisms facilitate biofortification, enriching crops with vital nutrients and fostering sustainable agricultural practices.

Biofortification is not a new concept, but its integration with soil microorganisms brings forth a nuanced understanding of the intricate relationships within ecosystems. As we navigate the challenges posed by climate change and a burgeoning global population, the significance of sustainable agriculture becomes paramount. Soil microorganisms, through their diverse functionalities, become instrumental allies in achieving the delicate balance between increased food production and environmental stewardship. In acknowledging the imperative of biofortification, this chapter sheds light on the specific roles played by soil microorganisms in nutrient enhancement (Khan et al., 2019). Nitrogen-fixing bacteria, for instance, have the capacity to convert atmospheric nitrogen into a form readily usable by plants, thus bolstering their growth and protein content. Similarly, phosphate-solubilizing fungi contribute to improved phosphorus uptake, a critical element for various biochemical processes in plants. The synthesis of plant growth-promoting substances further fortifies crops against environmental stressors, enhancing their overall nutritional profile (Tripathi et al., 2022). As we explore the mechanisms employed by soil microorganisms, it becomes evident that their contributions extend beyond nutrient provision. The rhizosphere, enriched by the activities of these microorganisms, becomes a haven for plant health. The intricate network of interactions contributes to disease suppression, stress tolerance, and overall resilience in crops. In essence, the integration of soil microorganisms into agricultural practices goes beyond a mere nutrient boost; it cultivates a holistic and resilient agroecosystem (Singh and Prasanna, 2020).

The significance of microbial biofertilizers and biopesticides as viable alternatives to conventional agrochemicals further underscores the ecological benefits of incorporating soil microorganisms into agricultural strategies. The reduction of chemical inputs not only mitigates environmental risks but also fosters a more balanced and sustainable agricultural ecosystem. The positive feedback loop between soil health and crop productivity becomes apparent, emphasizing the need to transition towards practices that prioritize ecological harmony (Kaur et al., 2021). As we navigate the complexities of modern agriculture, the role of advanced biotechnological tools cannot be overstated. Metagenomics, a powerful approach to studying genetic material recovered directly from environmental samples, provides insights into the vast genomic diversity of soil microorganisms. Synthetic biology, with its capacity to design and engineer biological systems, opens new frontiers in tailoring microbial consortia for specific crops and environmental conditions. The convergence of these technologies offers a promising trajectory for optimizing biofortification strategies and ensuring their efficacy in diverse agroecosystems (Kaur et al., 2020).

This chapter aims to synthesize current knowledge, draw attention to successful case studies, and delineate the challenges and future directions in the realm of soil microorganisms and biofortification. By understanding the intricate interplay between soil microorganisms and plants, we pave the way for a sustainable agricultural future that addresses nutritional needs, preserves the environment, and fosters resilience in the face of global challenges.

7.2 SOIL MICROORGANISMS: THE DRIVERS OF NUTRIENT DYNAMICS

The intricate world beneath our feet, hidden from the naked eye, is teeming with life. Soil microorganisms, including bacteria, fungi, and archaea, form a diverse and dynamic community that plays a central role in nutrient cycling within the soil ecosystem, as shown in Figure 7.1. This section delves into the fascinating realm of soil microorganisms, exploring their diversity, functions, and the pivotal role they play as drivers of nutrient dynamics (Suman et al., 2022).

7.2.1 DIVERSITY OF SOIL MICROORGANISMS

The soil, often considered a complex matrix of minerals and organic matter, is, in fact, a bustling microbial metropolis. The microbial diversity in soil is staggering, with an estimated one gram of soil containing billions of microorganisms belonging to thousands of different species. Bacteria, the most numerous, are accompanied by fungi, archaea, viruses, and various microscopic animals, collectively forming a vibrant and interconnected web of life (Yang et al., 2021). This diversity is not just

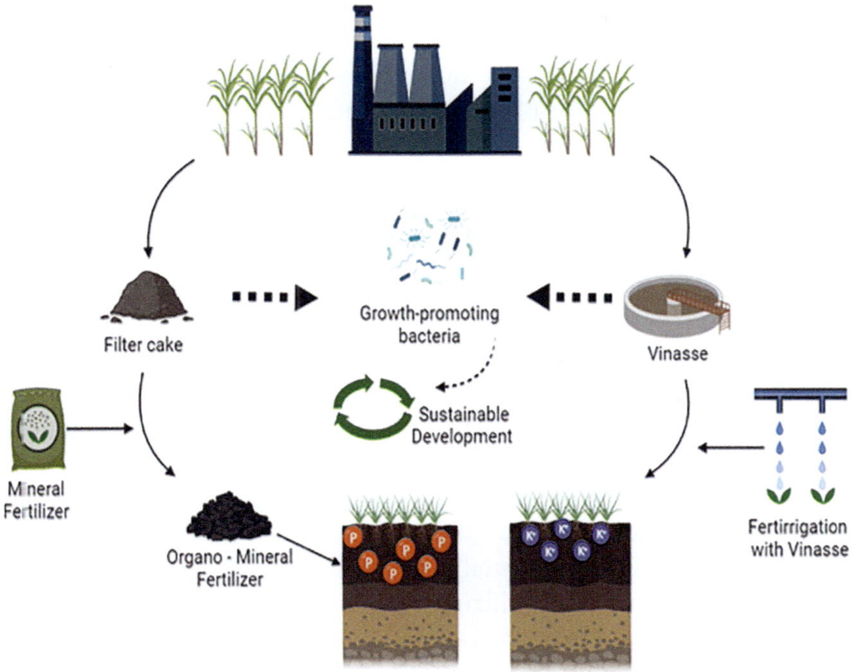

FIGURE 7.1 The captivating domain of soil microorganisms, highlighting their diversity and functions.

a testament to the richness of soil ecosystems but also a key factor in sustaining soil health. Different microorganisms contribute distinct functions, from decomposing organic matter to fixing nitrogen and aiding in nutrient mineralization. Understanding this microbial diversity is crucial for unraveling the complexities of nutrient dynamics within the soil.

7.2.2 THE RHIZOSPHERE: MICROBIAL HOTSPOT

Within the soil, the rhizosphere represents a microenvironment surrounding plant roots where the dynamic interplay between plants and soil microorganisms unfolds. Plant roots release a variety of organic compounds into the soil, a phenomenon known as rhizodeposition, which serves as a veritable feast for soil microorganisms (Hakim et al., 2021). This influx of organic matter creates a hotspot for microbial activity, influencing nutrient availability and uptake by plants. The rhizosphere, therefore, becomes a hub for nutrient transformations facilitated by soil microorganisms.

Bacteria and fungi, in particular, colonize the rhizosphere, forming symbiotic relationships with plant roots and influencing the nutrient status of the surrounding soil. The activities within this microenvironment have profound implications for plant health, growth, and ultimately, the nutritional content of crops (Hussain et al., 2018).

7.2.3 NUTRIENT CYCLING AND SOIL MICROORGANISMS

Soil microorganisms are the architects of nutrient cycling, orchestrating processes that transform organic and inorganic materials into forms that plants can readily absorb. Nitrogen, a fundamental element for plant growth, undergoes transformations facilitated by nitrogen-fixing bacteria. These microbes convert atmospheric nitrogen into ammonia, making it available for plant uptake. In a complementary role, other bacteria participate in nitrification, converting ammonia into nitrate, a form that plants can readily utilize (Singh et al., 2019).

Phosphorus, another essential nutrient, is made available through the activities of phosphate-solubilizing fungi. These fungi release enzymes that break down complex forms of phosphorus into soluble compounds, enhancing its accessibility to plants. The rhizosphere becomes a nexus of these nutrient transformations, where soil microorganisms act as catalysts for processes that sustain the soil nutrient pool (Vikas and Ranjan, 2023).

7.2.4 PLANT-MICROBE INTERACTIONS

The interactions between soil microorganisms and plant roots are nuanced and sophisticated. In addition to nutrient cycling, these interactions influence plant health, disease resistance, and stress tolerance. Certain bacteria, for example, act as biocontrol agents, suppressing soil-borne pathogens and enhancing plant resilience. Mycorrhizal fungi form mutualistic associations with plant roots, facilitating nutrient uptake in exchange for carbohydrates produced by the plant through photosynthesis (Yadav et al., 2019).

7.3 BIOFORTIFICATION MECHANISMS EMPLOYED BY SOIL MICROORGANISMS

In the intricate dance between soil microorganisms and plants, the mechanisms employed by these microbes play a crucial role in enhancing the nutritional content of crops (Mishra et al., 2023). This section explores the biofortification mechanisms employed by soil microorganisms, shedding light on how they contribute to the enrichment of crops with essential nutrients.

7.3.1 NITROGEN-FIXING BACTERIA: ENHANCING PLANT NITROGEN AVAILABILITY

One of the primary biofortification mechanisms involves nitrogen-fixing bacteria. Nitrogen, a key component of amino acids, proteins, and chlorophyll, is vital for plant growth. However, atmospheric nitrogen (N_2) is in a form that most plants cannot directly utilize. Nitrogen-fixing bacteria, commonly associated with the root nodules of leguminous plants, possess the remarkable ability to convert atmospheric nitrogen into a more accessible form – ammonia (NH_3) or ammonium ions (NH_4^+) (Chauhan et al., 2021). This conversion, known as nitrogen fixation, enhances the nitrogen content of the soil and facilitates its uptake by plants, as shown in Figure 7.2. The symbiotic relationship between these bacteria and certain plant species is a prime example of how soil microorganisms contribute to biofortification by increasing the nitrogen availability for crops (Motesharezadeh et al., 2020).

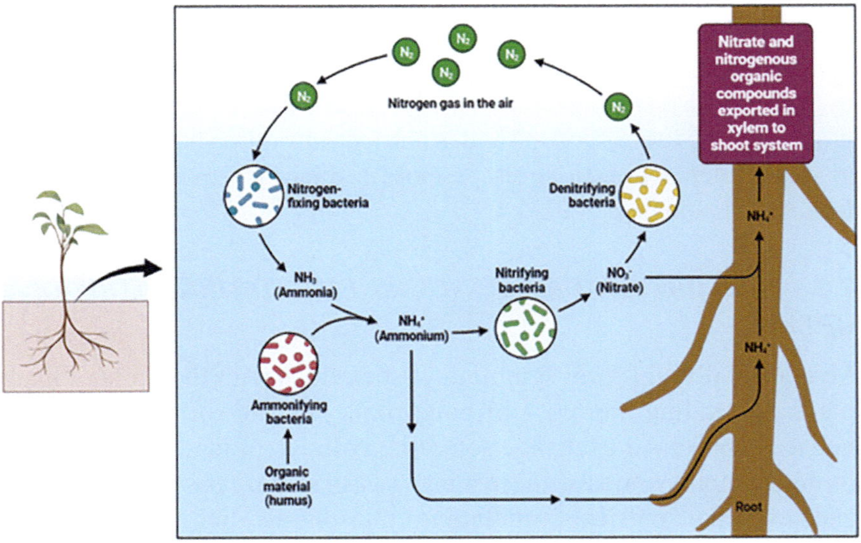

FIGURE 7.2 Nitrogen fixation: Types and mechanism.

7.3.2 PHOSPHATE-SOLUBILIZING FUNGI: IMPROVING PHOSPHORUS UPTAKE

Phosphorus is another essential nutrient critical for various biochemical processes in plants, including energy transfer, photosynthesis, and nucleic acid synthesis. However, phosphorus in the soil is often present in insoluble forms, making it less accessible to plants. Enter phosphate-solubilizing fungi (Chen and Liao, 2017). These fungi produce enzymes, such as phosphatases, that break down complex forms of phosphorus in the soil, converting them into soluble forms that plants can readily absorb. By enhancing phosphorus solubility, these fungi play a pivotal role in improving the phosphorus uptake efficiency of plants, contributing significantly to the biofortification of crops (Rehman et al., 2019).

7.3.3 PLANT GROWTH-PROMOTING SUBSTANCES: AIDING NUTRIENT ABSORPTION AND STRESS TOLERANCE

Beyond the direct provision of nutrients, soil microorganisms contribute to biofortification by synthesizing plant growth-promoting substances. These include hormones, enzymes, and other bioactive compounds that positively influence plant growth and development (Dubey et al., 2017). For instance, auxins produced by certain bacteria stimulate root development, increasing the surface area for nutrient absorption. Additionally, the production of siderophores by microorganisms enhances iron uptake by plants, addressing a common micronutrient deficiency. These growth-promoting substances not only aid in nutrient absorption but also contribute to stress tolerance, making crops more resilient to environmental challenges (Waseem et al., 2023).

7.3.4 MYCORRHIZAL ASSOCIATIONS: FACILITATING NUTRIENT UPTAKE

Mycorrhizal fungi form symbiotic associations with the roots of many plants, extending the reach of plant roots into the soil and enhancing nutrient uptake. In exchange for carbohydrates produced by the plant through photosynthesis, these fungi assist in the absorption of water and essential nutrients, including phosphorus and micronutrients (Adhikari et al., 2021). Arbuscular mycorrhizal fungi, in particular, are known to play a significant role in biofortification by improving the nutrient status of crops. The hyphal network formed by these fungi acts as an extension of the plant root system, exploring a larger soil volume and accessing nutrients that may be beyond the reach of the plant alone (Ray et al., 2020).

7.4 MICROBIAL BIOFERTILIZERS AND BIOPESTICIDES

In the ongoing quest for sustainable agriculture, the utilization of microbial biofertilizers and biopesticides represents a paradigm shift away from conventional chemical inputs. This section explores the significance, mechanisms, and applications of these biological tools, emphasizing their potential to enhance soil health, promote plant growth, and mitigate the environmental impacts associated with traditional agricultural practices (Upadhayay et al., 2019).

7.4.1 MICROBIAL BIOFERTILIZERS: NURTURING SOIL HEALTH

1. **Microbial Biofertilizers:** These encompass a diverse array of microorganisms, predominantly bacteria and fungi, deliberately introduced into the soil to enhance nutrient availability for plants. Unlike chemical fertilizers, which provide nutrients in soluble forms, microbial biofertilizers contribute to nutrient cycling and solubilization through biological processes (Thompson and Tschida, 2023).
2. **Nitrogen-Fixing Bacteria:** One of the key players in microbial biofertilizers is nitrogen-fixing bacteria. Species like *Rhizobium* and *Azotobacter* form symbiotic relationships with plants, particularly legumes, converting atmospheric nitrogen into a form (*ammonia*) that plants can readily use. This biological nitrogen fixation (BNF) not only enriches the soil with nitrogen but also promotes sustainable agricultural practices by reducing the need for synthetic nitrogen fertilizers (Kumar et al., 2022).
3. **Phosphate-Solubilizing Fungi:** In addition to nitrogen-fixers, phosphate-solubilizing fungi contribute significantly to microbial biofertilizers. Fungi like *mycorrhizae* release enzymes that break down insoluble forms of phosphorus in the soil, making it accessible to plants. This enhances phosphorus uptake efficiency, particularly in phosphorus-deficient soils, fostering improved plant growth and health (Igiehon and Babalola, 2017).

4. **Plant Growth-Promoting Substances:** Microbial biofertilizers also produce plant growth-promoting substances, such as auxins and cytokinin's. These substances stimulate root development, increase nutrient absorption, and enhance overall plant vigor. By fostering a more robust root system, microbial biofertilizers contribute to improved nutrient uptake and water utilization by plants (Tiwari et al., 2019).

7.4.2 BIOPESTICIDES: NAVIGATING TOWARDS SUSTAINABLE PEST MANAGEMENT

1. **Introduction to Biopesticides:** Biopesticides are formulations derived from living organisms or their byproducts, designed to control pests while minimizing environmental impact. In contrast to synthetic chemical pesticides, biopesticides leverage the inherent antagonistic relationships between microbes and pests, providing a sustainable alternative for pest management (Bhatt and Bhatt, 2021).
2. **Bacterial Biopesticides:** These utilize bacteria such as *Bacillus thuringiensis* (*Bt*), which produces toxins lethal to specific insect pests shown in Figure 7.3. These biopesticides are highly specific, targeting only the intended pests while sparing beneficial organisms. This selectivity minimizes ecological disruption, making them an environmentally friendly option for pest control (Lee et al., 2019).

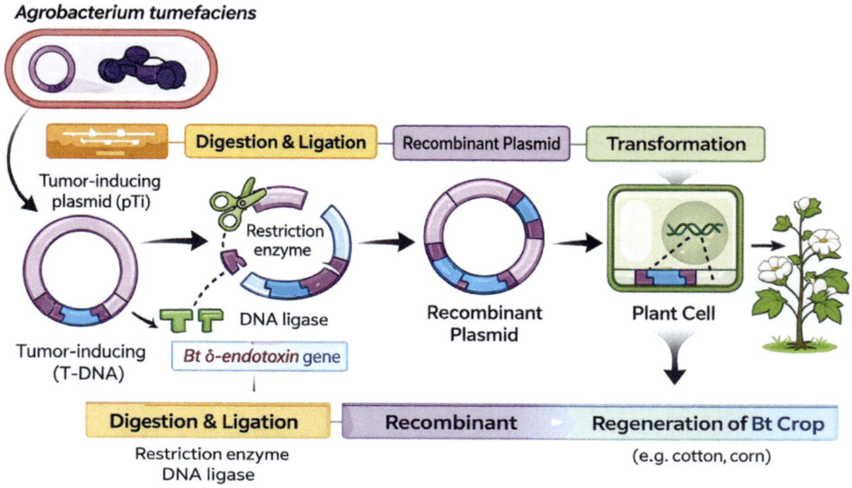

FIGURE 7.3 Transformation of crops with *Bacillus thuringiensis* (*Bt*).

3. **Fungal Biopesticides:** These often based on species like *Beauveria bassiana* and *Metarhizium anisopliae*, exploit the entomopathogenic properties of certain fungi. These fungi infect and parasitize insects, offering a natural and effective means of pest control. Fungal biopesticides are particularly valuable in integrated pest management (IPM) strategies, providing a sustainable alternative to chemical insecticides (Backer et al., 2018).

4. **Benefits of Biopesticides:** Biopesticides offer several advantages, including a reduced environmental footprint, lower toxicity to non-target organisms, and decreased likelihood of pest resistance development. Moreover, they align with the principles of IPM, emphasizing a holistic approach that combines biological, cultural, and mechanical control methods (Bano et al., 2021).

7.5 ECOLOGICAL IMPLICATIONS AND SOIL HEALTH

The health of soil is intricately linked to the broader ecological dynamics of a given environment. This section explores the ecological implications of soil health, emphasizing the pivotal role of soil microorganisms in maintaining ecosystem balance, fostering biodiversity, and contributing to the overall sustainability of terrestrial ecosystems (Lewis, 2021).

1. **Microbial Diversity in the Soil:** Soil is a habitat rich in microbial life, hosting an immense diversity of bacteria, fungi, archaea, and other microorganisms. This diversity is not only a testament to the complexity of soil ecosystems but also a key indicator of soil health. Different microorganisms play distinct roles in nutrient cycling, organic matter decomposition, and the formation of symbiotic relationships with plants (Basavegowda and Baek, 2021).

2. **Symbiotic Relationships and Plant Diversity:** Symbiotic associations between soil microorganisms and plants contribute significantly to both soil health and plant diversity. Mycorrhizal fungi, for example, form mutualistic relationships with the roots of many plants, enhancing nutrient uptake and supporting plant growth (Patel et al., 2020). This, in turn, contributes to the overall diversity of plant species in an ecosystem.

7.5.1 NUTRIENT CYCLING AND ECOSYSTEM PRODUCTIVITY

1. **Soil Microorganisms as Nutrient Cyclers:** Soil microorganisms, especially bacteria and fungi, are key players in nutrient cycling. Nitrogen-fixing bacteria convert atmospheric nitrogen into forms usable by plants, contributing to nitrogen cycling. Phosphate-solubilizing fungi enhance phosphorus availability, supporting nutrient cycling. These microbial activities are fundamental for sustaining the productivity of terrestrial ecosystems (Freitas and Silva, 2022).

2. **Organic Matter Decomposition:** Decomposition of organic matter by soil microorganisms is a cornerstone of nutrient cycling. Microorganisms break down complex organic compounds into simpler forms, releasing nutrients that are then available for plant uptake. This process not only enriches the soil with essential nutrients but also supports the development of healthy plant communities (Roriz et al., 2020).

7.5.2 SOIL STRUCTURE AND WATER REGULATION

1. **Microbial Contributions to Soil Structure:** Soil structure, influenced by microbial activities, is crucial for water retention, aeration, and root penetration. Microorganisms produce substances like glues and polysaccharides, which bind soil particles together, creating aggregates that improve soil structure. Well-structured soils enhance water infiltration, reduce erosion, and provide a conducive environment for plant roots (Ijaz et al., 2023).

2. **Water Regulation and Erosion Prevention:** Healthy soils, enriched by the activities of soil microorganisms, play a vital role in water regulation. They act as reservoirs, holding water during periods of excess and releasing it during dry spells. This regulation helps prevent waterlogging and contributes to resilience in the face of changing weather patterns. Moreover, the binding effects of microorganisms on soil particles reduce the risk of erosion, preserving the integrity of ecosystems (Steinhoff-Knopp et al., 2021).

7.5.3 RESILIENCE AND SUSTAINABLE ECOSYSTEMS

1. **Microbial Roles in Resilience:** Soil microorganisms contribute to the resilience of ecosystems in the face of environmental stressors. Plant-microbe interactions, such as those involving mycorrhizal fungi, enhance the ability of plants to withstand drought, pathogens, and other challenges (Philippot et al., 2021). This resilience, fostered by the diverse and dynamic microbial communities in the soil, is a key component of ecosystem sustainability.
2. **Sustainable Agriculture and Soil Health:** The ecological implications of soil health extend to agricultural systems. Sustainable agriculture, which prioritizes soil health, incorporates practices that support biodiversity, nutrient cycling, and water regulation. By harnessing the natural functions of soil microorganisms, sustainable agriculture strives to balance the need for increased food production with environmental conservation (Usharani et al., 2019).

7.6 MODERN BIOTECHNOLOGICAL APPROACHES

Modern biotechnological approaches have revolutionized agriculture, offering innovative solutions to enhance crop productivity, improve nutritional content, and address environmental challenges. This section explores the cutting-edge techniques and tools that fall under the umbrella of modern biotechnology, focusing on their applications in agriculture (Atieno et al., 2020).

1. **Metagenomics: Unraveling Microbial Diversity:** Metagenomics involves the study of genetic material recovered directly from environmental samples, providing insights into the genomic diversity of entire microbial communities. In agriculture, metagenomics is employed to unravel the complexities of microbial populations in soil, the rhizosphere, and other agroecosystems. Metagenomics enables the identification of diverse microbial species and their functional capacities (Sousa et al., 2022). This information is crucial for understanding the roles of soil microorganisms in nutrient cycling, plant-microbe interactions, and overall soil health. By deciphering the genetic makeup of

microbial communities, researchers can design targeted interventions to optimize soil fertility and enhance plant performance.

2. **Synthetic Biology: Designing Tailored Microbial Consortia:** Synthetic biology involves the design and engineering of biological systems for specific purposes. In agriculture, synthetic biology is applied to create tailored microbial consortia with enhanced capabilities, such as nutrient fixation, biocontrol, and stress tolerance. By manipulating the genetic components of microorganisms, synthetic biology allows the creation of designer microbes optimized for agricultural goals (Che and Men, 2019). For example, researchers can engineer nitrogen-fixing bacteria to increase nitrogen fixation rates or enhance the production of plant growth-promoting substances. These custom-designed microbial consortia can be applied to crops, contributing to biofortification, disease resistance, and overall sustainable agricultural practices.

3. **CRISPR-Cas9: Precision Genome Editing:** CRISPR-Cas9 is a revolutionary genome editing tool that allows precise modification of specific genes. In agriculture, CRISPR-Cas9 is used to enhance crop traits, improve resistance to diseases, and optimize nutritional content. CRISPR-Cas9 enables targeted modifications in the genomes of crops, leading to the development of genetically modified organisms (GMOs) with desired traits (Wada et al., 2020). This tool has been used to create crops with increased resistance to pests and diseases, improved tolerance to environmental stresses, and enhanced nutritional profiles. CRISPR technology offers a more precise and efficient method of genetic modification, allowing for the development of crops with improved performance and sustainability (Molla and Yang, 2020).

4. **Precision Agriculture: Integrating Data and Technology:** Precision agriculture involves the use of technology, data analytics, and biotechnology to optimize farm management practices. It utilizes information from sensors, satellite imagery, and biotechnological tools to tailor agricultural practices to specific conditions. Precision agriculture integrates biotechnological approaches to monitor and manage crop conditions with high precision (Torky and Hassanein, 2020). For example, sensors can detect nutrient levels in the soil, and based on this information, automated systems can

deliver precise amounts of fertilizers. This approach minimizes resource inputs, reduces environmental impact, and maximizes crop yield, showcasing the synergy between modern biotechnology and precision agriculture.

7.6.1 CHALLENGES AND FUTURE DIRECTIONS IN AGRICULTURAL BIOTECHNOLOGY

The field of agricultural biotechnology has witnessed remarkable advancements, but it also faces challenges that require thoughtful consideration. This section delves into the current challenges and envisions future directions for agricultural biotechnology, exploring the path forward to harness its full potential for sustainable and resilient food production.

7.6.2 CHALLENGES IN AGRICULTURAL BIOTECHNOLOGY

1. **Public Perception and Acceptance:** GMOs and other biotechnological interventions often face skepticism and concerns from the public regarding safety, ethics, and environmental impact. Resistance to biotechnological applications can impede their adoption and hinder the realization of their benefits in agriculture (Rastegari et al., 2020).
2. **Regulatory Hurdles:** Stringent and sometimes inconsistent regulatory frameworks across countries can slow down the development and commercialization of biotechnological innovations (Khan et al., 2019). Cumbersome regulatory processes may impede the timely introduction of new technologies to address pressing agricultural challenges.
3. **Ethical Considerations:** Questions of equity, ethical use of technology, and potential impacts on small-scale farmers must be carefully addressed to ensure that biotechnological advancements benefit all segments of society. Unresolved ethical concerns may lead to unequal access to the benefits of agricultural biotechnology.
4. **Biodiversity and Ecological Impact:** The introduction of genetically modified crops and other biotechnological interventions may have unintended consequences on biodiversity and ecosystem

dynamics (Hussain et al., 2018). Ecological disruptions could affect pollinators, non-target organisms, and the overall resilience of ecosystems.

5. **Emergence of Resistance:** Pests, diseases, and weeds may evolve resistance to genetically modified crops or biotechnological pest control methods over time. Resistance could reduce the efficacy of these technologies, necessitating continuous innovation to stay ahead of evolving challenges.

7.6.3 FUTURE DIRECTIONS IN AGRICULTURAL BIOTECHNOLOGY

1. **Gene Editing Advancements:** Continued advancements in gene editing technologies, such as CRISPR-Cas9, hold immense potential for precise and targeted genetic modifications. Improved precision allows for the development of crops with enhanced traits, reduced off-target effects, and faster development timelines (Ijaz et al., 2023).

2. **Synthetic Biology Innovations:** Synthetic biology will play a pivotal role in designing customized microorganisms and pathways to optimize plant-microbe interactions, nutrient cycling, and stress tolerance. Tailored microbial consortia with specific functions can contribute to sustainable agriculture, addressing challenges related to soil health and nutrient availability (Atieno et al., 2020).

3. **Data-Driven Agriculture:** Integrating biotechnology with data analytics and artificial intelligence can lead to more efficient and precise farming practices under the umbrella of precision agriculture. Smart farming technologies can enhance resource-use efficiency, reduce environmental impact, and optimize crop management strategies.

4. **Climate-Resilient Crops:** Biotechnological approaches can be harnessed to develop crops with enhanced resilience to climate change, including tolerance to extreme temperatures, drought, and salinity. Climate-resilient crops are essential for ensuring food security in the face of changing environmental conditions (Lewis, 2021).

5. **Public Engagement and Education:** Fostering transparent communication, public engagement, and educational initiatives are crucial for building trust and addressing concerns related to biotechnological applications in agriculture. Informed public discourse can lead to more balanced perspectives on the benefits and risks associated with agricultural biotechnology.

6. **Global Collaboration:** Encouraging international collaboration in research, development, and regulatory frameworks can accelerate the responsible and equitable deployment of biotechnological solutions. Collaborative efforts can pool expertise, resources, and diverse perspectives, addressing challenges on a global scale.

7.6.4 NAVIGATING THE FUTURE OF AGRICULTURAL BIOTECHNOLOGY

As agricultural biotechnology continues to evolve, addressing challenges and charting future directions is paramount for realizing its potential in sustainable and resilient food production. Balancing scientific innovation with ethical considerations, engaging the public in informed discussions, and fostering global collaboration will be instrumental in steering agricultural biotechnology towards a future where it contributes significantly to addressing global food security challenges while respecting environmental and societal concerns (Thompson and Tschida, 2023).

7.7 CONCLUSION

In the pursuit of sustainable agriculture, the role of soil microorganisms in biofortification strategies and ecological implications becomes increasingly evident. The intricate dance between these unseen allies and the agricultural ecosystem unveils a promising avenue for addressing global challenges related to food security, malnutrition, and environmental sustainability. The utilization of soil microorganisms for biofortification stands as a cornerstone in the pursuit of sustainable agriculture. From nitrogen-fixing bacteria enriching the soil with plant-available nitrogen to phosphate-solubilizing fungi enhancing phosphorus uptake, the mechanisms employed by these microorganisms offer nature-inspired solutions to nutrient deficiencies. This approach not only bolsters the nutritional content of crops but also aligns with the principles of ecological balance and resilience. The rhizosphere emerges as a microcosm of ecological harmony, where plant roots and soil microorganisms engage in intricate interactions. This hotspot of biological activity contributes to nutrient cycling, disease suppression, and overall soil health. As we harness the potential of these interactions, the ecological implications extend beyond crop yield to encompass the development of robust and resilient agroecosystems.

However, as with any transformative endeavor, challenges emerge on the path to harnessing soil microorganisms for sustainable agriculture. Balancing the need for increased food production with environmental conservation, addressing public concerns, and navigating regulatory landscapes pose hurdles that require careful consideration. Yet, within these challenges lie opportunities for innovation, education, and global collaboration. Looking ahead, the integration of modern biotechnological approaches, such as metagenomics and synthetic biology, holds promise for unraveling the mysteries of plant-microbe interactions and tailoring microbial consortia for optimized biofortification. The precision and efficiency of these tools offer a glimpse into a future where sustainable agriculture is not only an aspiration but a reality shaped by the strategic deployment of soil microorganisms. Biofortification strategies, coupled with an understanding of ecological implications, offer a nuanced pathway that goes beyond mere crop enhancement. It speaks to the resilience of ecosystems, the health of our soils, and the well-being of our communities. As we navigate the complexities of a changing climate and a growing global population, the significance of soil microorganisms becomes increasingly paramount. Their role in sustainable agriculture is not merely a scientific endeavor but a testament to the interconnectedness of all life on Earth. In embracing this synergy, we pave the way for a future where agriculture is not only a source of sustenance but a harmonious coexistence with the natural world. In the soil beneath our feet lies the foundation for a more sustainable and nourished planet, and through the harnessing of soil microorganisms, we cultivate the seeds of a resilient agricultural future.

KEYWORDS

- **agricultural ecosystem**
- **biofortification**
- **biotechnology**
- **climate-resilient crops**
- **metagenomics**
- **soil microorganisms**
- **sustainable agriculture**

REFERENCES

Adhikari, A., Pandey, K., Pant, V., Bisht, T. S., & Punetha, H. (2021). Biofortification of plants by using microbes. In *Microbial Technology for Sustainable Environment* (pp. 141–166).

Atieno, M., Herrmann, L., Nguyen, H. T., Phan, H. T., Nguyen, N. K., Srean, P., & Lesueur, D. (2020). Assessment of biofertilizer use for sustainable agriculture in the Great Mekong Region. *Journal of Environmental Management*, *275*, 111300.

Backer, R., Rokem, J. S., Ilangumaran, G., Lamont, J., Praslickova, D., Ricci, E., & Smith, D. L. (2018). Plant growth-promoting rhizobacteria: Context, mechanisms of action, and roadmap to commercialization of bio stimulants for sustainable agriculture. *Frontiers in Plant Science*, 1473.

Bano, S., Wu, X., & Zhang, X. (2021). Towards sustainable agriculture: Rhizosphere microbiome engineering. *Applied Microbiology and Biotechnology*, 1–20.

Basavegowda, N., & Baek, K. H. (2021). Current and future perspectives on the use of nano fertilizers for sustainable agriculture: The case of phosphorus nano fertilizer. *3 Biotech*, *11*(7), 357.

Bhatt, K., & Bhatt, P. (2021). Rhizosphere biology: Alternate tactics for enhancing sustainable agriculture. In *Phyto Microbiome Interactions and Sustainable Agriculture* (pp. 164–186).

Chauhan, A., Saini, R., & Sharma, J. C. (2021). Plant growth promoting rhizobacteria and their biological properties for soil enrichment and growth promotion. *Journal of Plant Nutrition*, *45*(2), 273–299.

Che, S., & Men, Y. (2019). Synthetic microbial consortia for biosynthesis and biodegradation: Promises and challenges. *Journal of Industrial Microbiology and Biotechnology*, *46*(9–10), 1343–1358.

Chen, L., & Liao, H. (2017). Engineering crop nutrient efficiency for sustainable agriculture. *Journal of Integrative Plant Biology*, *59*(10), 710–735.

Daly, D. H., Velivelli, S. L., & Prestwich, B. D. (2017). The role of soil microbes in crop biofortification. In *Agriculturally Important Microbes for Sustainable Agriculture: Volume I: Plant-Soil-Microbe Nexus* (pp. 333–356).

Dhiman, K., Sharma, D., Kumari, R., & Tomar, P. (2023). Biofortification of crops using microbes–A promising sustainable agriculture strategy. *Journal of Plant Nutrition, 46*(12), 2912–2935.

Dubey, R. K., Tripathi, V. T. V., Edrisi, S. A., Bakshi, M. B. M., Dubey, P. K., Singh, A. S. A., & Abhilash, P. C. (2017). Role of plant growth-promoting microorganisms in sustainable agriculture and environmental remediation. In *Advances in PGPR Research* (pp. 75–125). Wallingford UK: CABI.

Freitas, J., & Silva, P. (2022). Sustainable agricultural systems for fruit orchards: The influence of plant growth-promoting bacteria on the soil biodiversity and nutrient management. *Sustainability, 14*(21), 13952.

Hakim, S., Naqqash, T., Nawaz, M. S., Laraib, I., Siddique, M. J., Zia, R., & Imran, A. (2021). Rhizosphere engineering with plant growth-promoting microorganisms for agriculture and ecological sustainability. *Frontiers in Sustainable Food Systems, 5*, 617157.

Hussain, A., Zahir, Z. A., Asghar, H. N., Ahmad, M., Jamil, M., Naveed, M., & Zaman Akhtar, M. F. U. (2018). Zinc solubilizing bacteria for zinc biofortification in cereals: A step toward sustainable nutritional security. In *Role of Rhizosphere Microbes in Soil: Volume 2: Nutrient Management and Crop Improvement* (pp. 203–227).

Igiehon, N. O., & Babalola, O. O. (2017). Biofertilizers and sustainable agriculture: Exploring arbuscular mycorrhizal fungi. *Applied Microbiology and Biotechnology, 101*, 4871–4881.

Ijaz, S., Iqbal, J., Abbasi, B. A., Tufail, A., Ullah, Z., Sharifi-Rad, J., & Uddin, S. (2023). Biofortification: Lessons from the past and strategies for future food security. In *Legumes Biofortification* (pp. 521–545). Cham: Springer International Publishing.

Jaiswal, D. K., Krishna, R., Chouhan, G. K., de Araujo Pereira, A. P., Ade, A. B., Prakash, S., & Verma, J. P. (2022). Bio-fortification of minerals in crops: Current scenario and future prospects for sustainable agriculture and human health. *Plant Growth Regulation, 98*(1), 5–22.

Kaur, T., Devi, R., Kour, D., Yadav, A., Yadav, A. N., Dikilitas, M., & Saxena, A. K. (2021). Plant growth-promoting soil microbiomes and their potential implications for agricultural and environmental sustainability. *Biologia, 76*(9), 2687–2709.

Kaur, T., Rana, K. L., Kour, D., Sheikh, I., Yadav, N., Kumar, V., & Saxena, A. K. (2020). Microbe-mediated biofortification for micronutrients: Present status and future challenges. In *New and Future Developments in Microbial Biotechnology and Bioengineering* (pp. 1–17). Elsevier.

Khan, A., Singh, J., Upadhayay, V. K., Singh, A. V., & Shah, S. (2019). Microbial biofortification: A green technology through plant growth promoting microorganisms. In *Sustainable Green Technologies for Environmental Management* (pp. 255–269).

Kumar, A., Beura, K., & Singh, M. (2022). Micronutrient management in soils and the route to biofortification. In *Soil Management for Sustainable Agriculture* (pp. 379–401). Apple Academic Press.

Lee, S. K., Lur, H. S., & Liu, C. T. (2021). From lab to farm: Elucidating the beneficial roles of photosynthetic bacteria in sustainable agriculture. *Microorganisms, 9*(12), 2453.

Lewis, E. (2021). Biofortification as a sustainable solution for 'hidden hunger': Evaluating its impact on the environment, nutrition, culture, and ethics.

Mishra, P., Mishra, J., & Arora, N. K. (2023). Biofortification revisited: Addressing the role of beneficial soil microbes for enhancing trace elements concentration in staple crops. *Microbiological Research*, 127442.

Molla, K. A., & Yang, Y. (2020). Predicting CRISPR/Cas9-induced mutations for precise genome editing. *Trends in Biotechnology*, *38*(2), 136–141.

Motesharezadeh, B., Ghorbani, S., & Alikhani, H. A. (2020). The effect of selenium biofortification in alfalfa (*Medicago sativa*). *Journal of Plant Nutrition*, *43*(2), 240–250.

Patel, P., Trivedi, G., Bhatt, S., Patel, H., & Saraf, M. (2020). Development of sustainable biofortification strategy in *Phraseolus vulgaris* through selenorhizobacteria under selenium deficient region. *Biosciences Biotechnology Research Communications*, *13*, 1–9.

Philippot, L., Griffiths, B. S., & Langenheder, S. (2021). Microbial community resilience across ecosystems and multiple disturbances. *Microbiology and Molecular Biology Reviews*, *85*(2), 10–1128.

Rastegari, A. A., Yadav, A. N., & Yadav, N. (2020). *New and Future Developments in Microbial Biotechnology and Bioengineering: Trends of Microbial Biotechnology for Sustainable Agriculture and Biomedicine Systems: Diversity and Functional Perspectives*. Elsevier.

Ray, P., Lakshmanan, V., Labbé, J. L., & Craven, K. D. (2020). Microbe to microbiome: A paradigm shift in the application of microorganisms for sustainable agriculture. *Frontiers in Microbiology*, *11*, 622926.

Rehman, H. M., Cooper, J. W., Lam, H. M., & Yang, S. H. (2019). Legume biofortification is an underexploited strategy for combatting hidden hunger. *Plant, Cell & Environment*, *42*(1), 52–70.

Roriz, M., Barros, M., Castro, P. M., Carvalho, S. M., & Vasconcelos, M. W. (2020). Improving iron nutrition in plant foods: The role of legumes and soil microbes. In *Vitamins and Minerals Biofortification of Edible Plants* (pp. 103–122).

Roriz, M., Carvalho, S. M., Castro, P. M., & Vasconcelos, M. W. (2020). Legume biofortification and the role of plant growth-promoting bacteria in a sustainable agricultural era. *Agronomy*, *10*(3), 435.

Singh, D. P., Prabha, R., Renu, S., Sahu, P. K., & Singh, V. (2019). Agrowaste bioconversion and microbial fortification have prospects for soil health, crop productivity, and eco-enterprising. *International Journal of Recycling of Organic Waste in Agriculture*, *8*, 457–472.

Singh, D., & Prasanna, R. (2020). Potential of microbes in the biofortification of Zn and Fe in dietary food grains. A review. *Agronomy for Sustainable Development*, *40*, 1–21.

Sousa, J., Silvério, S. C., Costa, A. M., & Rodrigues, L. R. (2022). Metagenomic approaches as a tool to unravel promising biocatalysts from natural resources: Soil and water. *Catalysts*, *12*(4), 385.

Steinhoff-Knopp, B., Kuhn, T. K., & Burkhard, B. (2021). The impact of soil erosion on soil-related ecosystem services: Development and testing a scenario-based assessment approach. *Environmental Monitoring and Assessment*, *193*(Suppl 1), 274.

Suman, J., Rakshit, A., Ogireddy, S. D., Singh, S., Gupta, C., & Chandrakala, J. (2022). Microbiome as a key player in sustainable agriculture and human health. *Frontiers in Soil Science*, *2*, 821589.

Thompson, P., & Tschida, K. (2023). Microbial biofortification: A sustainable solution to feed 10 billion people. *Celebrating Scholarship and Creativity Day (2018–)*, 230. https://digitalcommons.csbsju.edu/ur_cscday/230 (accessed on 2nd January 2026).

Tiwari, S., Prasad, V., & Lata, C. (2019). *Bacillus*: Plant growth promoting bacteria for sustainable agriculture and environment. In *New and Future Developments in Microbial Biotechnology and Bioengineering* (pp. 43–55). Elsevier.

Torky, M., & Hassanein, A. E. (2020). Integrating blockchain and the internet of things in precision agriculture: Analysis, opportunities, and challenges. *Computers and Electronics in Agriculture*, *178*, 105476.

Tripathi, S., Bahuguna, R. N., Shrivastava, N., Singh, S., Chatterjee, A., Varma, A., & Jagadish, S. K. (2022). Microbial biofortification: A sustainable route to grow nutrient-rich crops under changing climate. *Field Crops Research*, *287*, 108662.

Upadhayay, V. K., Singh, J., Khan, A., Lohani, S., & Singh, A. V. (2019). Mycorrhizal mediated micronutrients transportation in food-based plants: A biofortification strategy. In *Mycorrhizosphere and Pedogenesis* (pp. 1–24).

Usharani, K. V., Roopashree, K. M., & Naik, D. (2019). Role of soil physical, chemical and biological properties for soil health improvement and sustainable agriculture. *Journal of Pharmacognosy and Phytochemistry*, *8*(5), 1256–1267.

Vikas, & Ranjan, R. (2023). Biofertilizers and biofortification in future agriculture. In *Climate-Resilient Agriculture, Vol 1: Crop Responses and Agroecological Perspectives* (pp. 363–377). Cham: Springer International Publishing.

Wada, N., Ueta, R., Osakabe, Y., & Osakabe, K. (2020). Precision genome editing in plants: State-of-the-art in CRISPR/Cas9-based genome engineering. *BMC Plant Biology*, *20*, 1–12.

Waseem, M., Aslam, M. M., Idris, A. L., Nkurikiyimfura, O., & Di, Z. (2023). Plant–microbe interaction for legume biofortification: Present status and future challenges. In *Legumes Biofortification* (pp. 271–293). Cham: Springer International Publishing.

Yadav, R., Ror, P., Rathore, P., & Ramakrishna, W. (2020). Bacteria from native soil in combination with arbuscular mycorrhizal fungi augment wheat yield and biofortification. *Plant Physiology and Biochemistry*, *150*, 222–233.

Yang, D., Hu, C., Wang, X., Shi, G., Li, Y., Fei, Y., & Zhao, X. (2021). Microbes: A potential tool for selenium biofortification. *Metallomics*, *13*(10), https://doi.org/10.1093/mtomcs/mfab054.

CHAPTER 8

Utilization of Beneficial Microorganisms for Nematode Management: Role in Sustainable Agriculture

PRITI PAL,[1] PRAKASH KUMAR SARANGI,[2]
AKHILESH KUMAR SINGH,[3] BRIJESH PANDEY,[3]
UTTAM KUMAR SAHOO,[4] and ANAND PRAKASH[3,*]

[1]*Amity Institute of Biotechnology, Amity University Uttar Pradesh, Lucknow Campus, Lucknow, India*

[2]*College of Agriculture, Central Agricultural University, Imphal, Manipur, India*

[3]*Department of Biotechnology, School of Life Sciences, Mahatma Gandhi Central University, Motihari, Bihar, India*

[4]*Department of Forestry, Mizoram University, Aizawl, Mizoram, India*

*Corresponding authors

ABSTRACT

Nematodes pose a significant threat to global agriculture, causing substantial yield losses and economic damage. Traditional nematode management strategies often rely on chemical nematicides, which raise environmental and health concerns. In the pursuit of sustainable agriculture, there is a growing interest in harnessing the potential of beneficial microorganisms for nematode management. This abstract explores the role of beneficial microorganisms, including bacteria, fungi, and nematophagous organisms, in mitigating nematode-induced crop damage while promoting sustainable agricultural practices. This abstract reviews recent advances in the identification, isolation,

Biotechnology for Sustainable Agriculture: Innovative Approaches and Strategies.
Prakash Kumar Sarangi (Ed)

DOI: 10.1201/9781779642998-8

and application of beneficial microorganisms for nematode management. It highlights successful case studies where the implementation of microbial-based strategies has demonstrated efficacy in reducing nematode populations and improving crop yields. The abstract concludes by emphasizing the need for continued research, innovation, and collaboration to unlock the full potential of beneficial microorganisms in promoting sustainable nematode management and ensuring global food security.

8.1 INTRODUCTION

Nematodes, those minuscule denizens of the soil, quietly wreak havoc on global agriculture, causing significant crop losses and economic distress. The conventional response to their insidious presence has long been dominated by chemical nematicides. However, the environmental and health concerns associated with these synthetic agents have prompted a reevaluation of nematode management strategies. In this transformative era, attention has shifted towards harnessing the innate power of beneficial microorganisms—bacteria, fungi, and hematophagous organisms—as a sustainable alternative (Devi and Devi, 2023). To understand the prowess of these microorganisms in nematode management, one must explore the intricate mechanisms at play in this microcosmic battlefield. From direct parasitism to the production of nematocidal compounds, the diversity of strategies employed by these micro-organisms forms a nuanced and sustainable approach to pest control (Soares et al., 2023). Beneficial bacteria invade nematode tissues, disrupting essential processes, while certain fungi release enzymes and toxins, creating a hostile environment (Devi et al., 2020). These mechanisms collectively constitute a microbial arsenal for nematode suppression. Recent advances in molecular biology and biotechnology have enabled the identification and isolation of nematode-suppressive microorganisms (Ney et al., 2019). Metagenomics and next-generation sequencing have unveiled the microbial diversity within soil ecosystems, shedding light on key players in the nematode management drama. By deciphering the genetic code of these microorganisms, researchers can tailor their application for maximum efficacy in nematode-infested soils (Fabiyi et al., 2023). Real-world successes underscore the triumphs of microbial-based nematode management strategies. From nematode-trapping fungi in organic farming to plant growth-promoting rhizobacteria in conventional agriculture, these case studies highlight the versatility and efficacy of microbial solutions across different agricultural landscapes (Rambal, 2021). Beyond nematode suppression, microbial-based strategies contribute to soil health, biodiversity preservation, and overall ecosystem balance, aligning seamlessly with the principles of sustainable agriculture. The symbiotic symphony between beneficial microorganisms and plants extends beyond the soil, stimulating the production of defense-related compounds within plants (Boni et al., 2023). This synergy creates a holistic approach to nematode management, enhancing the resilience of crops to infestations. However, the practical implementation of microbial-based strategies is not without challenges. Formulation, application methods, and environmental considerations require careful navigation to bridge the gap between theoretical potential and practical application. As we stand at the cusp of a microbial odyssey in nematode management, the imperative for continued research, innovation, and collaboration becomes apparent. The full potential of beneficial microorganisms in nematode control is yet to be fully unlocked (Musbau et al., 2021). By pushing the boundaries of knowledge, addressing challenges, and embracing opportunities, we can pave the way for a future where sustainable agriculture is not just an aspiration but a tangible reality. In doing so, we embark on a journey towards global food security, environmental stewardship, and a harmonious coexistence between agriculture and nature (Figure 8.1).

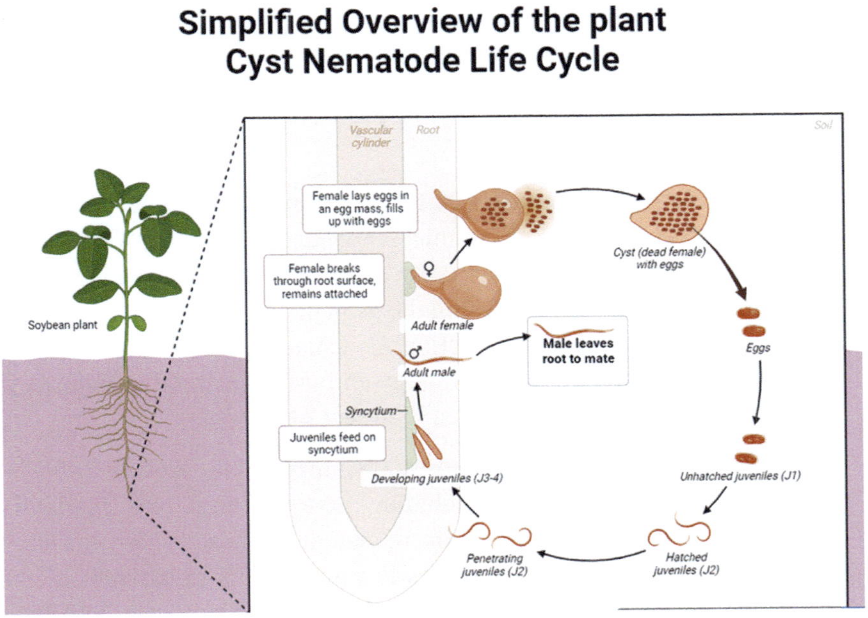

FIGURE 8.1 Life cycle of nematode in agriculture crop.

Source: Microbe notes. https://microbenotes.com/soybean-cyst-nematode/.

8.2 MECHANISMS OF ACTION

The mechanisms of action employed by beneficial microorganisms in nematode management are diverse and intricate, representing a micro-cosmic battlefield where these microscopic entities engage in a silent but strategic war against nematodes (Singh et al., 2023). Understanding these mechanisms is crucial for appreciating the multifaceted role of beneficial microorganisms in sustainable agriculture.

1. **Parasitism: Direct Invasion of Nematode Tissues:** Beneficial microorganisms, particularly certain bacteria and fungi, exhibit a parasitic lifestyle by directly invading nematode tissues. These microorganisms enter the nematode body, disrupting essential physiological processes and ultimately leading to the death of the nematode. This form of biological control serves as a direct and lethal method to suppress nematode populations (Gachara et al., 2023).
2. **Competition for Resources: Creating an Unfavorable Environment:** Beneficial microorganisms compete with nematodes for essential resources, such as nutrients and space within the soil ecosystem. By outcompeting nematodes for these resources, microorganisms create an inhospitable environment for nematode survival. This competitive exclusion weakens nematode populations, limiting their ability to proliferate and cause damage to crops (Elnahal et al., 2022).
3. **Production of Nematocidal Compounds: Chemical Warfare:** Some beneficial microorganisms are adept at producing secondary metabolites with nematicidal properties. These compounds act as natural pesticides, inhibiting the growth, development, or survival of nematodes. The production of nematicidal compounds represents a chemical warfare strategy employed by microorganisms to fend off nematode attacks and protect plant roots.
4. **Predation: Nematophagous Organisms in Action:** Nematophagous organisms, including certain fungi and predatory nematodes, actively prey on nematodes. These organisms have evolved specialized structures or mechanisms to capture, infect, and consume nematodes. By incorporating nematodes into their life cycle, nematophagous organisms contribute to the biological control of nematode populations in the soil.

5. **Induction of Plant Defenses: Symbiotic Interaction with Plants:** Beneficial microorganisms engage in symbiotic interactions with plants, stimulating the host plants to activate their innate defense mechanisms. This symbiosis results in the production of defense-related compounds within plants, making them more resilient to nematode infestations. The enhanced plant defenses contribute to a holistic approach to nematode management, promoting the overall health and vigor of crops (Kaur et al., 2023).

These mechanisms collectively form the arsenal of beneficial microorganisms in their endeavor to manage nematode populations. Importantly, the diversity of strategies allows for a dynamic and adaptable response to varying environmental conditions and nematode species. The intricate interplay between microorganisms and nematodes represents a sophisticated example of biological control in action, offering a sustainable and environmentally friendly alternative to traditional chemical-based nematode management strategies.

8.3 IDENTIFICATION AND ISOLATION OF BENEFICIAL MICROORGANISMS

The identification and isolation of beneficial microorganisms for nematode management involve advanced techniques in molecular biology, microbiology, and biotechnology. This process is crucial for understanding the specific characteristics and traits of these microorganisms, allowing researchers to harness their potential for sustainable agricultural practices. Here is an overview of the key steps and methodologies involved:

1. **Metagenomics: Unraveling Microbial Diversity:** Metagenomics is a powerful tool that allows researchers to study the genetic material (DNA or RNA) extracted directly from environmental samples, such as soil. In the context of nematode management, metagenomics provides insights into the microbial diversity present in the soil ecosystem. By analyzing the collective genetic material, researchers can identify a wide range of microorganisms, including bacteria, fungi, and other potential nematode antagonists (Ahirwar et al., 2020).

2. **Next-Generation Sequencing (NGS): Decoding the Genetic Blueprint:** Next-generation sequencing technologies have revolutionized the field of genomics by enabling the rapid and high-throughput sequencing of DNA. In the context of identifying beneficial microorganisms, NGS plays a pivotal role in decoding the genetic blueprint of the microbial communities present in soil samples. This technology allows researchers to uncover the specific genes, functions, and metabolic pathways that contribute to the nematode-suppressive capabilities of certain microorganisms.

3. **Isolation Techniques: Culturing and Characterization**: While metagenomics provides a comprehensive overview of microbial diversity, isolating individual microorganisms is essential for in-depth studies and practical application. Researchers use various culture-based techniques to isolate and grow individual strains of bacteria, fungi, or nematophagous organisms from soil samples. These isolates can then be characterized based on their morphological, physiological, and genetic traits.

4. **Functional Screening: Assessing Nematode-Suppressive Abilities:** Once isolated, microorganisms are subjected to functional screening to assess their nematode-suppressive abilities. This involves exposing nematodes to the isolated microorganisms under controlled laboratory conditions. Researchers observe and measure parameters such as nematode mortality, inhibition of nematode egg hatching, or reduction in nematode populations. This screening process helps identify the most effective nematode antagonists among the isolated microorganisms.

5. **Genetic and Molecular Techniques: Targeted Analysis:** Advanced genetic and molecular techniques are employed to delve deeper into the specific mechanisms and traits of isolated microorganisms. This includes the analysis of specific genes associated with nematode suppression, the production of nematicidal compounds, or other relevant traits. Polymerase chain reaction (PCR), gene expression analysis, and genomic sequencing contribute to a targeted understanding of the genetic basis of nematode antagonism.

6. **Bioinformatics: Data Analysis and Integration:** Bioinformatics plays a crucial role in analyzing the vast amounts of data generated through metagenomics and genomic sequencing. Computational tools and bioinformatic analyses help identify potential genes, pathways, and interactions that contribute to nematode management. This integrated approach enhances the understanding of the functional capacities of beneficial microorganisms (Hezakiel et al., 2023).

The identification and isolation of beneficial microorganisms for nematode management represent a multidisciplinary approach that combines molecular biology, microbiology, and computational biology. These techniques collectively provide researchers with the tools to uncover the microbial players in soil ecosystems, understand their genetic makeup, and harness their potential for sustainable agriculture.

8.3.1 CASE STUDIES: SUCCESS STORIES IN MICROBIAL NEMATODE MANAGEMENT

Case studies offer tangible examples of successful applications of microbial nematode management strategies in diverse agricultural settings. These success stories showcase the efficacy and versatility of utilizing beneficial microorganisms to mitigate nematode-induced crop damage. Here are a few illustrative examples:

1. **Nematode-Trapping Fungi in Organic Farming:** In organic farming systems, the application of nematode-trapping fungi has shown significant promise. Fungi such as *Arthrobotrys* and *Duddingtonia* have the ability to form adhesive structures, called traps, which capture and immobilize nematodes. By introducing these fungi into the soil, farmers can harness a natural and sustainable mechanism for suppressing nematode populations. The success of such applications lies in the ability of these fungi to adapt to diverse soil conditions and effectively target nematodes.
2. **Plant Growth-Promoting Rhizobacteria (PGPR) in Conventional Agriculture:** Plant growth-promoting rhizobacteria, commonly referred to as PGPR, have proven effective in conventional agriculture for nematode management. Certain strains of PGPR, such as species within the genera Bacillus and

Pseudomonas, establish symbiotic relationships with plant roots. These bacteria release compounds that not only stimulate plant growth but also induce systemic resistance against nematodes. This systemic defense mechanism enhances the plant's ability to withstand nematode attacks, resulting in improved crop yields.

3. **Arbuscular Mycorrhizal Fungi (AMF) in Sustainable Cropping Systems:** Arbuscular mycorrhizal fungi form mutualistic associations with plant roots, promoting nutrient uptake and enhancing plant tolerance to various stresses, including nematode infestations. Sustainable cropping systems that integrate the application of AMF have demonstrated success in managing nematode populations. The mycorrhizal network created by these fungi facilitates communication between plants, enabling them to share resources and activate defense mechanisms. This holistic approach contributes to sustainable nematode control while promoting soil health (Figure 8.2).

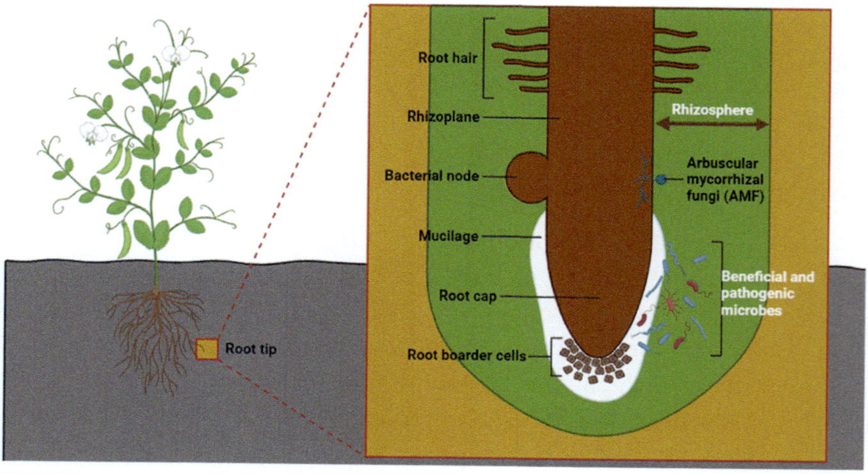

FIGURE 8.2 Arbuscular mycorrhizal fungi (AMF) in sustainable cropping systems: Enhancing soil health and crop resilience.

4. **Nematode-Bacterial Symbiosis for Crop Protection:** Certain beneficial bacteria establish symbiotic relationships with nematodes, offering a unique approach to nematode management. For example, *Xenorhabdus* and *Photorhabdus* are bacteria that

form mutualistic associations with entomopathogenic nematodes (EPNs). These nematodes seek out and infect insect *larvae*, releasing the bacteria, which then produce toxins lethal to the insects. Researchers have explored the potential of these bacteria in suppressing plant-parasitic nematodes, showcasing the adaptability of microbial strategies across different nematode-host systems.

5. **Combination Approaches for Enhanced Efficacy:** Some case studies highlight the synergistic effects of combining multiple beneficial microorganisms for enhanced nematode management. Integrating nematode-trapping fungi with plant growth-promoting rhizobacteria or mycorrhizal fungi, for instance, creates a multifaceted approach that addresses nematodes at different stages of their life cycle. These combination strategies demonstrate the potential for developing integrated pest management (IPM) systems that maximize efficacy while minimizing environmental impact (Paravar et al., 2023).

These case studies collectively underscore the success of microbial nematode management strategies in diverse agricultural contexts. The adaptability of beneficial microorganisms, their compatibility with different cropping systems, and their ability to integrate into existing agricultural practices contribute to the growing body of evidence supporting the feasibility and sustainability of microbial-based approaches in nematode control.

8.3.2 PROMOTION OF SUSTAINABLE AGRICULTURAL PRACTICES

The promotion of sustainable agricultural practices through the utilization of beneficial microorganisms in nematode management represents a paradigm shift away from conventional, chemical-intensive approaches. This shift aligns with broader principles of sustainable agriculture, emphasizing environmental stewardship, soil health, and long-term ecosystem resilience (Gupta et al., 2022). Here are key aspects illustrating how the use of beneficial microorganisms contributes to the promotion of sustainable agricultural practices:

1. **Reduced Reliance on Synthetic Pesticides:** One of the central tenets of sustainable agriculture is the reduction of reliance on

synthetic pesticides. The use of chemical nematicides can have detrimental effects on non-target organisms, disrupt soil ecosystems, and contribute to pesticide resistance. Beneficial microorganisms offer a natural and targeted alternative, mitigating the need for synthetic chemicals and minimizing their adverse environmental impact.

2. **Enhanced Soil Health:** Beneficial microorganisms contribute to the enhancement of soil health, a cornerstone of sustainable agriculture. These microorganisms play crucial roles in nutrient cycling, organic matter decomposition, and the maintenance of soil structure. By fostering a diverse and thriving soil microbiome, the use of beneficial microorganisms promotes soil fertility and resilience, creating an environment conducive to sustainable crop production (Swami, 2020).

3. **Preservation of Biodiversity:** Sustainable agriculture emphasizes the importance of biodiversity in maintaining resilient ecosystems. The application of beneficial microorganisms, particularly those that naturally occur in soil ecosystems, supports biodiversity by promoting the presence of diverse microbial communities. This, in turn, has cascading effects on other soil-dwelling organisms, contributing to a balanced and biodiverse agricultural landscape (Aguilar-Marcelino et al., 2020).

4. **Conservation of Beneficial Insects:** Certain beneficial microorganisms, such as those forming symbiotic relationships with EPNs, contribute to the conservation of beneficial insects. These microorganisms specifically target harmful insect pests while sparing non-target organisms. This targeted approach aligns with sustainable pest management practices that seek to preserve beneficial insects, essential for pollination and maintaining ecological balance.

5. **Mitigation of Environmental Impact:** The use of beneficial microorganisms in nematode management minimizes the environmental impact associated with conventional nematicides. Chemical nematicides can leach into water bodies, contaminate soil, and harm non-target organisms. In contrast, microbial-based strategies offer a more ecologically friendly solution, reducing

the risk of environmental pollution and fostering a harmonious coexistence between agriculture and the surrounding ecosystem (Musbau et al., 2021).

6. **Climate Resilience:** Sustainable agriculture aims to build climate-resilient farming systems capable of withstanding climate variability. Beneficial microorganisms contribute to climate resilience by improving soil structure, enhancing water retention, and aiding plants in adapting to stress conditions (Verma et al., 2019). These microorganisms contribute to the overall robustness of agricultural ecosystems in the face of changing climate patterns.
7. **Economic Viability for Farmers:** Sustainable agricultural practices are not only environmentally friendly but also economically viable for farmers. Beneficial microorganisms, once established in the soil, can contribute to long-term nematode management, reducing the need for repeated applications of synthetic nematicides (Usharani et al., 2020). This can lead to cost savings for farmers while maintaining or improving crop yields.

8.3.3 ENHANCEMENT OF PLANT DEFENSE MECHANISMS

Beyond direct nematode suppression, beneficial microorganisms play a role in enhancing plant defense mechanisms. This section explores how the interaction between microorganisms and plants can stimulate the production of defense-related compounds, bolstering the resilience of crops to nematode infestations.

8.3.4 CHALLENGES AND OPPORTUNITIES

Implementing microbial-based nematode management strategies presents a spectrum of challenges and opportunities, intricately woven into the fabric of sustainable agriculture. Navigating this terrain requires a holistic understanding of the complexities involved.

1. **Challenges:**

   i. **Formulation Complexity:** Crafting formulations that maintain the viability and efficacy of beneficial microorganisms poses a challenge. Developing stable formulations that can be easily applied in diverse agricultural settings requires careful consideration of factors such as shelf life, compatibility, and ease of application.

ii. **Application Methods:** Determining optimal application methods for beneficial microorganisms can be challenging. Factors like soil type, climate, and crop variety influence the effectiveness of microbial application. Developing practical and efficient delivery mechanisms that ensure even distribution throughout the soil profile is an ongoing challenge.

iii. **Environmental Considerations:** The environmental fate of applied microorganisms is a critical concern. Factors such as temperature, moisture, and the presence of antagonistic microorganisms in the soil can impact the survival and activity of beneficial strains. Balancing environmental considerations while optimizing microbial efficacy is a complex challenge.

iv. **Scaling Up Production:** The large-scale production of beneficial microorganisms for widespread agricultural use presents logistical and economic challenges. Achieving consistent and cost-effective production to meet the demands of diverse farming operations requires addressing issues related to scalability and production efficiency.

v. **Integration into Farming Systems:** Integrating microbial-based nematode management into existing farming practices can be met with resistance or skepticism from farmers accustomed to conventional methods. Bridging the gap between scientific innovation and on-the-ground implementation necessitates effective knowledge transfer, extension services, and farmer education (Seenivasagan and Babalola, 2021).

2. **Opportunities:**

i. **Innovation in Formulation Technology:** Advances in formulation technology present opportunities to enhance the stability and efficacy of beneficial microorganisms. Novel formulations, such as encapsulation techniques or carrier materials, offer the potential to address challenges related to shelf life and ease of application.

ii. **Precision Agriculture:** The advent of precision agriculture technologies provides an opportunity to tailor the application of beneficial microorganisms to specific areas within a field. Precision agriculture enables the optimization of microbial distribution, maximizing their impact on nematode populations while minimizing resource use.

iii. **Biotechnology and Genetic Engineering:** Ongoing advancements in biotechnology and genetic engineering open avenues for customizing microorganisms to enhance their nematode-suppressive traits. Tailoring microorganisms for specific soil conditions or nematode species offers the potential to optimize their efficacy in diverse agricultural environments (Yadav and Sarkar, 2019).

iv. **Collaborative Research and Extension Services:** Collaboration between researchers, agricultural extension services, and farmers is essential for successful implementation. Building collaborative networks fosters the exchange of knowledge, addresses challenges in real-world contexts, and facilitates the adoption of microbial-based strategies on a broader scale.

v. **Market Development for Microbial Products:** The growing interest in sustainable agriculture creates opportunities for the development of a robust market for microbial-based products. Increased awareness, coupled with supportive policies and incentives, can drive market growth, making microbial solutions more accessible to farmers (Devki et al., 2021).

vi. **Resilience and Adaptability:** Beneficial microorganisms exhibit resilience and adaptability to diverse environmental conditions. Harnessing these traits presents an opportunity to develop microbial-based solutions that are effective across a range of agroecosystems and climates (Poveda and Eugui, 2022).

In navigating the challenges and opportunities associated with microbial-based nematode management, researchers, farmers, and industry stakeholders play pivotal roles in shaping the trajectory of sustainable agriculture. Addressing challenges creatively and capitalizing on opportunities is essential for realizing the full potential of these microbial strategies in promoting resilient and environmentally friendly farming practices.

8.3.5 FUTURE DIRECTIONS AND CONCLUDING REMARKS

The future of microbial-based nematode management lies in a trajectory of continual research, innovation, and practical implementation. As we conclude our exploration of these sustainable strategies, it is crucial to reflect on the evolving landscape and potential pathways that will shape the integration of beneficial microorganisms into global agriculture. Future research will likely witness advancements in microbial genomics, offering a deeper understanding of the genetic mechanisms underlying nematode suppression. This knowledge will enable the identification and engineering of microbial strains with enhanced efficacy, adaptability, and specificity for nematode control (Manetsberger et al., 2023). The exploration of synergistic effects within microbial consortia will be a focal point. Combining multiple strains of beneficial microorganisms with complementary traits could result in enhanced nematode suppression and increased resilience to environmental variations. The concept of precision agriculture will extend to microbial applications, utilizing technologies such as remote sensing and data analytics to tailor the distribution of beneficial microorganisms with precision. This approach optimizes resource utilization and maximizes the impact on nematode populations. Future research efforts will delve into comprehensive ecological and environmental impact assessments of microbial-based nematode management (Cha et al., 2021). Understanding the long-term effects on soil health, non-target organisms, and overall ecosystem dynamics will be crucial for sustainable implementation. The integration of microbial strategies with other sustainable agricultural practices, such as cover cropping, organic farming, and agroecological approaches, will be explored. Synergies between these practices may amplify the benefits of microbial nematode management within holistic farming systems. Collaborative efforts between researchers, policymakers, farmers, and industry stakeholders will strengthen the global knowledge base. Establishing platforms for knowledge sharing, collaborative research projects, and international cooperation will accelerate the adoption of microbial-based strategies on a broader scale.

In conclusion, the utilization of beneficial microorganisms for nematode management signifies a promising era in sustainable agriculture. As we navigate challenges and seize opportunities, these microbial strategies offer a nuanced and environmentally friendly alternative to conventional nematicides. The journey towards sustainable agriculture involves a collective commitment to ongoing research, technological innovation, and the translation of scientific knowledge into practical solutions for farmers. By fostering a symbiotic relationship between scientific inquiry and on-the-ground application, we can envision a future where microbial-based nematode management is seamlessly integrated into diverse agricultural landscapes. Recognizing the interconnectedness of agriculture, ecology, and global food security is essential. The potential of beneficial microorganisms extends beyond nematode management, contributing to the broader goals of resilience, biodiversity conservation, and environmental sustainability. In the coming years, the convergence of scientific ingenuity, technological advancements, and collaborative efforts will shape the landscape of sustainable agriculture. By embracing the potential of beneficial microorganisms, we pave the way for a future where agriculture not only meets the demands of a growing population but does so in a manner that is ecologically conscious, economically viable, and socially responsible.

KEYWORDS

- **global agriculture**
- **microbial strategies**
- **microorganisms**
- **nematode**
- **sustainable agricultural practices**
- **symbiotic relationship**

REFERENCES

Aguilar-Marcelino, L., Mendoza-de-Gives, P., Al-Ani, L. K. T., López-Arellano, M. E., Gómez-Rodríguez, O., Villar-Luna, E., & Reyes-Guerrero, D. E. (2020). Using molecular techniques applied to beneficial microorganisms as biotechnological tools for controlling agricultural plant pathogens and pest. In *Molecular Aspects of Plant Beneficial Microbes in Agriculture* (pp. 333–349). Academic Press.

Ahirwar, N. K., Singh, R., Chaurasia, S., Chandra, R., & Ramana, S. (2020). Effective role of beneficial microbes in achieving the sustainable agriculture and eco-friendly environment development goals: A review. *Frontiers in Microbiology, 5*, 111–123.

Beni, S. B., Mlowe, N., & Swai, T. (2023). Influence of effective micro-organisms in vegetable production: The case of two climatic zones in Tanzania. In *1st Kagera Annual Agricultural Conference and Exhibitions (KAACE).*

Cha, B. K., Pandeya, B., Chanda, H., Bhusala, P., Pandita, S., & Khanalb, S. (2021). Promotion of organic and sustainable agriculture through the use of biofertilizers. *Journal of Wastes and Biomass Management (JWBM), 3*(1), 01–08.

Devi, M. M., & Devi, K. D. (2023). Role of micro-organism for improving soil health. *Sustainable Management of Soil Health, 7.*

Devi, T. S., Das, D., Ansari, R. A., Rizvi, R., Sumbul, A., & Mahmood, I. (2020). Role of organic additives in the sustainable management of Phyto parasitic nematodes. In *Management of Phytonematodes: Recent Advances and Future Challenges* (pp. 279–295).

Devki, D. N., Sudan, J., & Kumar, D. (2021). Advances in microbes use in agricultural biotechnology. In *Crop Improvement: Biotechnological Advances* (p. 237).

Elnahal, A. S., El-Saadony, M. T., Saad, A. M., Desoky, E. S. M., El-Tahan, A. M., Rady, M. M., & El-Tarabily, K. A. (2022). The use of microbial inoculants for biological control, plant growth promotion, and sustainable agriculture: A review. *European Journal of Plant Pathology, 162*(4), 759–792.

Fabiyi, O. A., Adebisi, O. O., Falore, S. O., & Claudius-Cole, A. O. (2023). Potential inhibition of entomopathogenic nematodes and plant growth-promoting bacteria with exposure to selected herbicides and insecticides. *Vegetos*, 1–10.

Gachara, G., Kenfaoui, J., Suleiman, R., Kilima, B., Taoussi, M., Aberkani, K., & Lahlali, R. (2023). The role of soil microbiome in driving plant performance: An overview based on ecological and ecosystem advantages to the plant community. *Gesunde Pflanzen*, 1–15.

Gupta, R., Anand, G., Pandey, R., & Yadav, D. (2022). Microbial management of Phyto nematode in medicinal and aromatic plants: An eco-friendly approach.

Hezakiel, H. E., Thampi, M., Rebello, S., & Sheikhmoideen, J. M. (2023). Biopesticides: A green approach towards agricultural pests. *Applied Biochemistry and Biotechnology*, 1–30.

Kaur, H., Hussain, S. J., Mir, R. A., Verma, V. C., Naik, B., Kumar, P., & Dubey, R. C. (2023). Nano fertilizers–emerging smart fertilizers for modern and sustainable agriculture. *Biocatalysis and Agricultural Biotechnology, 102921.*

Manetsberger, J., Caballero Gómez, N., Soria-Rodríguez, C., Benomar, N., & Abriouel, H. (2023). Simply versatile: The use of *Peribacillus simplex* in sustainable agriculture. *Microorganisms, 11*(10), 2540.

Musbau, S. A., Ayinde, B. H., Omowunmi, O. O., Motunrayo, E. L., Belay, E., Teshome, B., & Sarwar, M. T. (2021). Micro and macro (organisms) and their contributions to soil fertility. *Frontiers in Environmental Microbiology, 7*, 44.

Ney, L., Franklin, D., Mahmud, K., Cabrera, M., Hancock, D., Habteselassie, M., & Subedi, A. (2019). Sensitivity of nematode community analysis to agricultural management practices and inoculation with local effective microorganisms in the Southeastern United States. *Soil Systems, 3*(2), 41.

Paravar, A., Piri, R., Balouchi, H., & Ma, Y. (2023). Microbial seed coating: An attractive tool for sustainable agriculture. *Biotechnology Reports, e00781.*

Poveda, J., & Eugui, D. (2022). Combined use of *Trichoderma* and beneficial bacteria (mainly *Bacillus* and *Pseudomonas*): Development of microbial synergistic bio-inoculants in sustainable agriculture. *Biological Control, 105100.*

Rambal, K. (2021). Impact of fungal inoculants on sustainable agriculture. In *Fungi Bio-Prospects in Sustainable Agriculture, Environment and Nano-Technology* (pp. 189–202). Academic Press.

Seenivasagan, R., & Babalola, O. O. (2021). Utilization of microbial consortia as biofertilizers and biopesticides for the production of feasible agricultural product. *Biology, 10*(11), 1111.

Singh, D., Devi, K. B., Ashoka, P., Bahadur, R., Kumar, N., Devi, O. R., & Shahni, Y. S. (2023). Green manure: Aspects and its role in sustainable agriculture. *International Journal of Environment and Climate Change, 13*(11), 39–45.

Soares, C. R. F. S., Hernández, A. G., Da Silva, E. P., De Souza, J. E. A., Bonfim, D. F., Zabot, G. L., & Brunetto, G. (2023). Applications and market of micro-organism-based and plant-based inputs in Brazilian agriculture. *Plants, 12*(22), 3844.

Swami, S. (2020). Soil microbes for securing the future of sustainable farming. *International Journal of Current Microbiology and Applied Sciences, 9*, 2687–2706.

Usharani, K. V., Roopashree, K. M., & Naik, D. (2019). Role of soil physical, chemical and biological properties for soil health improvement and sustainable agriculture. *Journal of Pharmacognosy and Phytochemistry, 8*(5), 1256–1267.

Verma, D. K., Pandey, A. K., Mohapatra, B., Srivastava, S., Kumar, V., Talukdar, D., & Asthir, B. (2019). Plant growth-promoting rhizobacteria: An eco-friendly approach for sustainable agriculture and improved crop production. In *Microbiology for Sustainable Agriculture, Soil Health, and Environmental Protection* (pp. 3–80). Apple Academic Press.

Yadav, K. K., & Sarkar, S. (2019). Biofertilizers, impact on soil fertility and crop productivity under sustainable agriculture. *Environment and Ecology, 37*(1), 89–93.

CHAPTER 9

Microbial Pathogens on Insect Pests for Sustainable Agriculture

PRABH NARAYAN MEENA,* DEVARAMANE RAGHAVENDRA, LICON KUMAR ACHARYA, M. K. KHOKHAR, and SUBHASH CHANDER

ICAR–National Research Center for Integrated Pest Management, Pusa Campus, New Delhi, Delhi, India

*Corresponding authors

ABSTRACT

The judicious application of chemical pesticides in agriculture in near past has led to environmental contamination; natural enemies' disturbance, pesticide resistance development among pests, outbreak of minor and secondary pest's and pest resurgence. Microbial bioagents like Fungi, virus, bacteria and nematodes etc. which are safe to humans and other non-targeted organisms have played pivotal role in replacing the pest pressure created by chemical pesticides. Most extensively used insect pathogen is the bacteria, *Bacillus thuringiensis (Bt)* for the management of lepidopteran pests. *Bt kurstaki* a bacterial strain which was imported in India are very expensive and there is challenge to develop indigenous *Bt* strains which should be cheap and compatible to use against different crop pests. Among the entomopathogenic fungi like *Beauveria brongniartii, B. bassiana, Metarhizium anisopliae* var. *acridium, M. anisopliae, Lecanicillium* spp., *Hirsutella thompsonii, Isaria fumosorosea,* and *Nomuraea rileyi* are playing vital role in insect pest control in recent years. Besides, *Anticarsia gemmatalis* NPV in Brazil, *Lymantria dispar* and *Orgyia pseudotsugata* NPV in USA and GV of *Pieris rapae* are used in China. Entomopathogenic nematodes such as (*Steinernema* spp. and *Heterorhabditis* spp.) also getting more attention in controlling crop pests.

Biotechnology for Sustainable Agriculture: Innovative Approaches and Strategies.
Prakash Kumar Sarangi (Ed)

DOI: 10.1201/9781779642998-9

9.1 INTRODUCTION

Due to the increase in adverse effects of chemical pesticides, nowadays, research is considerably focusing on environmentally friendly microbial pathogens. Around 1.3% of the world's pesticide market is occupied by microbial biopesticides, the majority (90%) of them used as insecticides (Menn and Hall, 2001). The pathogens that cause disease in insects are fungi, bacteria, viruses, protozoans, and nematodes. The most successful and widely used insect pathogen is *Bacillus thuringiensis*, which occupies around 2% of the total pesticide market in the world (Bravo et al., 2011). Different subspecies or strains of *B. thuringiensis* produce a mix of toxins which are lethal to one or a few related insect species. For example, for lepidopteran larvae (*Bt* subspecies *kurstaki* and *aizawai*), for coleopteran larvae (*Bt* subspecies *tenebrionis*) and for mosquitoes (*Bt* subspecies *israelensis*). Among the EPF, like *Beauveria* spp., *Metarhizium* spp., *Lecanicillium* spp., and *Isaria* spp. are the most successful mycopesticides developed against various groups of insects (Faria and Wrait, 2007). Insect viruses, especially baculoviruses (NPV and Granulosis virus, GV) are most successful in controlling *Lepidoptera* and *Diptera* because of their specificity. NPVs are employed in the control of devastating pests (*Heliothis* spp. and *Spodoptera* spp.) in different countries on cotton, fruit, and vegetable crops (Rosell et al., 2008). Entomopathogenic nematodes (EPNs) are of substantial interest because of their possible use as biological control agents of a wide range of lepidopteran insects.

For the control of pests of agriculture and forestry, several hundreds of commercial products of bacteria, fungi, viruses, and nematodes are available worldwide. Success stories of large-scale control of insect pest species by microbial pathogens are the management of *Lymantria* spp. using the products of *B. thuringiensis* subspecies *kurstaki* (*Btk*), which was an outbreak in Poland and North America forests (Butt et al., 1999), management of Pine caterpillar with *B. bassiana* in China (Li et al., 2010), control of locusts in Africa, Australia, and China with *Metarhizium anisopliae* var. *acridium* (Lomer et al., 2001), sugarcane spittle bug management by *M. anisopliae* in Brazil, management of rubber lace bug with *Sporothrix insectorum*, control of corn borer with *B. bassiana* in Europe and USA (Rosell et al., 2008), and management of European pine sawfly with NPV in Europe and North America (Lord, 2005).

The major advantages of these microbial pathogens are that they are species-specific to target pests, safe to non-target organisms, do not cause adverse effects on the environment and human health, and they can be used against conventional insecticide-resistant pest populations.

9.1.1 BACILLUS THURINGIENSIS (BT)

Bacterial entomopathogens offer a variety of benefits, such as they can be used as stand-alone insecticides, in combination with chemical pesticides, and they can be employed in rotation. Most of the bacterial insect pathogens belong to the families Bacillaceae, Enterobacteriaceae, Pseudomonadaceae, Streptococcaceae, and Micrococcaceae. The majority of these are weak pathogens which infect insects during environmental stress, but a few are very virulent. The most important one is Bacillaceae. For example, milky disease in *scarabaeids* caused by *Bacillus popillae* and *Bacillus sphaericus* kills mosquitoes. The majority of bio-pesticides are bacterial based, because it is cheaper. Spore forming entomopathogenic bacteria, especially *B. thuringiensis* (*Bt*), have been extensively used for the control of insect pests of various agricultural crops. *Bt* (Cry toxins) is commercially available for use against different species of insect pests, that is, *Lepidoptera*, *Coleoptera*, and *Diptera*, and also for use through genetic engineering (*Bt* crops) against insect pests and weeds. The specificity of the toxins is resolute by molecular configuration, host midgut physiology, and toxin receptors present on midgut epithelium (Gill et al., 1992; Schnepf et al., 1998).

9.1.2 HISTORY OF BT

The first discovery of *Bt* in the world was done by the Japanese biologist Shigetane Ishiwatari, as that was killing silkworms, the causal organism for sotto disease (*Bacillus sotto*) (Milner, 1994). From a dead Mediterranean flour moth, Ernst Berliner isolated the same bacteria in Thuringia, Germany, in 1911 and named it *Bt*. Later, Berliner reported the existence of parasporal bodies near the endospore and called it a crystal in 1915. However, during 1956, Milner discovered the insecticidal activity of the parasporal crystal against lepidopteran insects (Milner, 1994). *Bt* was commercially produced and used under the name Sporine to kill flour moths during 1938 in France (Luthy et al., 1982). In the USA, commercialization of *Bt* was practiced during 1956, but due to poor-quality formulations, the products were not successful (Milner, 1994). Due to increased resistance to chemical pesticides by insects during the 1980s, the use of *Bt* was popularized worldwide (Milner, 1994).

9.1.3 THE CRYSTAL

Cry toxin (cry from crystal) formed during the sporulation process of *Bt* is called a crystal and referred to as insecticidal crystal protein, crystalline inclusion, delta endotoxin, or parasporal body. These cry toxins are species-specific to Hymenoptera, Lepidoptera, Diptera, Coleoptera, and Nematoda. These toxins are ineffective against vertebrates, humans, and predators and parasitoids of insect pests (Hofte and Whitely, 1989).

Bt israelensis produces cytolytic protein or Cyt toxin. Under *in vitro* conditions, the Cyt toxin is cytolytic to a vast group of invertebrate and vertebrate cells. These toxins are found to be more effective on dipteran (suborder: Nematocera) and coleopteran insects. Cyt toxin is also formed during the sporulation process and is present within the parasporal body but in a separate inclusion. Both have no significant amino acid sequence identity with Cry toxins (Hofte and Whitely, 1989). *Bt* toxins are listed in Jim Deacon (Table 9.1).

TABLE 9.1 *Bt* Toxins and Their Classification

Gene	Crystal Shape	Insect Activity
Cry I	Bipyramidal	Lepidoptera
Cry II	Cuboidal	Lepidoptera and Diptera
Cry III	Flat/irregular	Coleoptera
Cry IV	Bipyramidal	Diptera
Cry V-IX	Various	Various

9.2 MODE OF ACTION

Bacillus thuringiensis (*Bt*) is the most widely used insect pathogen present in soil and is lethal to caterpillars, beetles, flies, and so forth (Bahadur, 2018). *Bt* is a spore-forming, rod-shaped bacterium and is associated with the synthesis of crystal protoxin protein, which has insecticidal activity. After ingestion into the insect mid-gut, crystals dissolve in alkaline pH and are subsequently cleaved enzymatically by proteases of the host and form an active insecticidal toxin called δ-endotoxin (Cry proteins). The parasporal bodies (crystals) produced by these bacteria containing endotoxin (Cry proteins) act by ingestion through a pore-forming mechanism, which is detrimental to the gut epithelium of the insect (Pigott and Ellar, 2007).

Insects show different types of responses based on the type of cry proteins (δ-endotoxin). Responses showed by caterpillars to toxins are mentioned below (Dara, 2017).

- **Type 1 Response:** Within a few minutes after ingestion of toxins, mid-gut paralysis occurs. Symptoms include the insect stopping feeding, hemolymph pH increasing, vomiting starting, diarrhea, and becoming sluggish. After 24–48 hours, septicemia and general paralysis will occur, and the insect will die. Examples of Type-I response insects are tobacco hornworm, tomato hornworm, and silkworm.
- **Type 2 Response:** Midgut paralysis can be observed within a few minutes after ingestion of endotoxins, but no general paralysis will occur. After 48–72 hours, septicemia occurs. Examples of type II response insects are cabbage butterfly, alfalfa caterpillar, and inchworms.
- **Type 3 Response:** After ingestion of endotoxin in the insect body, midgut paralysis followed by cessation of feeding will occur. No symptoms of paralysis will be seen as insects move actively, and death of the insect can occur within 48–96 hours. Examples of insects include corn worm and gypsy moth.
- **Type 4 Response:** Insects are naturally resistant to infection; younger instars are most susceptible than older ones. After ingestion of endotoxins, mid-gut paralysis occurs, and the insect stops feeding. Insects move actively, and no general paralysis will occur. Insect mortality can be observed after 72–96 hours. Examples of this category of insects are armyworms and cutworms.

The type of response is different in mosquitoes, unlike caterpillars. The mosquito larva will die within 20–30 min after ingestion of *Bt* subsp. *Israelensis*.

1. **Mass Production:** *Bt* is the only microbial pest control agent that has been commercialized worldwide on a large scale. In India, *Bt* is freely available in the market, though it is still more expensive

compared to synthetic pesticides. Cost-effective methods of production and availability of native strains of *Bt* make it more valuable to farmers. The most widely used *Bt* species is *kurstaki*. Because it has no contact action and must be ingested to be effective, it should be applied to sites where larvae are feeding (Prasad et al., 2011).

2. **Production Procedure:** A small soil sample (1 g) is placed in 25 ml of 0.25 M sodium acetate solution in Luria broth and shaken for 2 hours. At the end, the sample is placed in a water bath at 80°C for 2 hours. All spore-forming bacteria germinate in sodium acetate, but not *Bt*. The heat shock kills the vegetative stages of all other bacteria. A loopful of the suspension is then streaked on L-agar medium. Colonies of *Bt* are picked with the help of a needle and transferred into the slants. After three days, the culture is observed for identification.

3. **Staining and Identification of *Bt*:** *Bt* isolates can be identified based on the presence of a parasporal or crystal body. For this, the *Bt* culture is grown on a synthetic medium, the spore + crystal mixture harvested, spread over a micro slide, and subjected to differential staining as described.

4. **Reagent A:** 5 g of Amido schwartz stain (Napthol blue black, buffalo black NBR, Amodo black are synonyms) is dissolved in 50 ml of 98% methanol, 40 ml water, and 10 ml acetic acid. Best results are obtained when the reagent is stored for 3 days after preparation.

5. **Reagent B (Ziehl's Carbol Fuschin):** 1 g basic Fuchsin is dissolved in 10 ml of 95% ethanol and mixed with 5 g of phenol dissolved in 90 ml of distilled water. It is to be used at 30% aqueous solution. A thin layer of Reagent A is pipetted over the heat-fixed *Bt* smears while the slide is still warm. After 70 seconds or so, the stain is washed off with cold tap water. While still wet, the smear is then covered with an even layer of Reagent B for 20 seconds, washed in cold tap water, and dried on filter paper. A standard blue filter is used in a light microscope. The slide is studied under immersion oil at 1000X. The presence of crystals, which look violet to dark blue, and spores, which look pink, confirm the presence of the isolate as *Bt*.

The same staining procedure is used during quality control of the product.

1. **Commercial Production:** The commercial production of *Bt* can be easily practiced on artificial synthetic medium by adopting conventional fermentation techniques either on the surface of semi-solid or submerged fermentation. In the former method, semi-solid media nutrients are contained in a coarse porous matrix with a large surface area. Humidity has to be maintained within narrow limits to allow growth. Semi-solid medium composed of 545 g wheat bran, 380 g expanded perlite, 62 g soybean meal, 36 g dextrose, 3.6 g lime, 0.9 g NaCl, 0.29 g $CaCl_2$ and 160 ml of water. After partial sterilization with steam for 60 minutes, the mixture weighs about 1.0 kg. This is inoculated with 400ml of fermented seed. At this time, 250 kg of bran medium is inoculated. The final product is the mixture of unutilized bran medium, spores, crystals, and other by-products of fermentation.

Although semi-solid media are difficult to sterilize, adjust the pH, and keep sterile during mass production and maintain uniform conditions. However, submerged culture is the preferred process for commercial mass production.

The submerged fermentation process involves a stepwise buildup of *Bt* cells. A liquid nutritive medium is used to suspend and propagate *Bt* biomass. Two such media nutritive compositions are given in Table 9.2.

TABLE 9.2 Nutritional Composition

Media A		**Media B**	
Ingredients	**Weight (g)**	**Ingredients**	**Weight (g)**
Tryptose	10.0	Profio*	1.0
Dextrose	5.0	Pepton	20.0
Starch	5.0	Dextrose	15.0
Yeast extract	2.0	Yeast extract	2.0
K_2HPO_4	1.0	$MgSO_4{\cdot}7H_2O$	0.30
KH_2PO	1.0	$FeSO_4{\cdot}7H_2O$	0.02
Double distilled water	1000 ml	$ZnSO_4{\cdot}H_2O$	0.02
		$CaCo_3$	1.0
		Double distilled water	1000

**Profio*: Partially defatted cooked cottonseed flour.

Carbon and nitrogen organic substances could be utilized after standardization of protocols. A typical *Bt* fermentation is started by inoculating a flask of culture medium with a loopful of bacterial colony on an agar plate. The flask is then incubated at 28°C on a shaker for spore germination and for proper adaptation of vegetative cells into the culture medium. After 10–16 hours, the cells are in mid-log phase. The culture is used to inoculate a 20-liter fermenter. Growth in the fermenter is again microscopically monitored until the spores start to lyse. During fermentation, antifoaming agents need to be added, and pH and oxygen supply monitored.

2. **Recovery:** The final contents of the fermenter must first be stabilized and screened to remove large debris comprising cells or growth medium. Initial screening may be done by ultra-filtration, screening, or centrifugation. The product is then processed by centrifugation or evaporation to increase the potency of the broth and form an aqueous concentrate. A spore count of $2–5*10^9$ spores/ml is obtained for the fermented product.
3. **Formulation:** The aqueous concentrate is then formulated as:
   i. Liquid suspension concentrates.
   ii. Wettable granules.
   iii. Wettable powder.
   iv. Oil flowable using a few additional steps (Table 9.3).

TABLE 9.3 Targeted Insect Pests by *B. thuringiensis* in Various Crops

SL. No.	Crop	Insect	Dosage (kg/ha)
1.	Cauliflower, cabbage	DMB, cabbage butterfly	0.5–1.50
2.	Brinjal	Stem borer, fruit borer	0.25–0.50
3.	Tomato, cotton, okra, chickpea, sunflower	Fruit borer	0.5–1.50
4.	Cauliflower, cabbage, cotton	Tobacco caterpillar	10.0

9.2.1 GENETIC ENGINEERING

To improve desired change in an organism, a gene should be transferred from another organism under laboratory conditions, called genetic engineering. Various gene transfer methods are available for plants and animals. One of the oldest and most traditional ways is selective breeding, in which a specific trait is identified and selected, and bred to produce more plants with the same traits. Nowadays, advanced technology offers the transfer of new traits from one plant to another under laboratory conditions (Martineau, 2011). One such example is *Bt* crops, which are genetically modified plants that contain *Bt* endotoxin, offering resistance to certain groups of insect pests. The first transgenic tobacco was produced by Plant Genetic Systems company in Belgium during 1985, but it was not very commercially successful. In 1995, the Environmental Protection Agency (EPA), USA, approved the production and distribution of transgenic crops (*Bt*) such as cotton, corn, potato, and tobacco (Vaek et al., 1987). At present, the most successful commercially cultivated transgenic crops in the world are cotton and corn. During 2013, Bangladesh approved four eggplants (*Bt brinjal*) for seed production and commercialization (Koch et al., 2015).

9.2.2 APPLICATION

During 1997, GM crops were cultivated worldwide in an area of 1.7 million ha, which gradually increased to 185.0 million ha during 2016 in 26 countries. There are five major transgenic crops viz., corn and cotton (insect resistant alone and insects and herbicide resistant), soybean, canola, and sugar beet (herbicide resistant) commercially cultivated worldwide. In the USA, the cultivated area of GM crops was 72.9 million ha (representing 39% of the world's total area), followed by Brazil (27%), Argentina (13%), Canada (6%), India (6%), Paraguay (2%), Pakistan (2%), China (2%), and South Africa (1%). In European countries, GM crops cultivated during 2015 covered about 117,000 ha, which increased to 136,000 ha in 2016 in countries viz., Spain, Portugal, Czech Republic, Slovakia, and Romania. During 2016, Romania did not plant GM crops due to difficult procedure requirements from the government (James, 2016). Commercially available *Bt* formulations (Ramanujam et al., 2014) available worldwide are listed in Table 9.4.

Even though *Bt* and its toxins are very effective as biopesticides in controlling various insect pests (List of *Bt* strains registered in India (Table 9.5)), excessive use can lead to the development of resistance. Diamondback moth, corn earworm, and tobacco budworm developed resistance to *Bt* toxins. Through genetic engineering, *Bt* toxins were inserted into various plants viz., cotton, corn, brinjal, potato, and soybean to protect

TABLE 9.4 Commercial *Bacillus thuringiensis* Formulations Available Worldwide

Manufacturer	Product	*Bt* Strain Employed	Target Pest(s)
Valent Biosciences Corporation	Dipel WP	*Bacillus thuringiensis*	Gypsy moth; bagworm; spring and cabbage looper
	Thuricide 48LV (liquid suspension)	*Bt*	Bagworm; elm worm; gypsy moth
	Novodor Flowable Concentrate	*Bt* ssp. *tenebrionis*	Colorado potato beetle; elm leaf beetle
	Foray 48B	–	–
	Foray 48B A (low volume)	–	Jack pine budworm; eastern hemlock looper
	Foray 76B (aqueous concentrate)	–	White-marked tussock moth; forest tent caterpillar; satin moth
AFA Environment Inc.	Aquabac II XT (liquid suspension)	*Bt israelensis* (*B. thuringiensis* serotype H-14)	Mosquitoes
	Aquabac 200G (10/14) (granules)	*Bt israelensis*	Mosquitoes
	Aquabac 200G (10/14) (5/8)	*Bt israelensis*	Mosquitoes
AFA Environment Inc.	Aquabac XT	*Bt israelensis*	Mosquitoes; blackflies
Abbott Lab. Ltd. (1988)	Dipel 176 (emulsifiable suspension)	–	Forest tent caterpillar; gypsy moth; spruce budworms; hemlock looper
AEF Global Inc.	Bioprotect (aqueous biological)	–	Gypsy moth; jack pine budworm; satin moth; white-marked tussock moth

against various pests, and there is a reduction in pesticide sprays. However, there is a need for suitable management approaches necessary to reduce *Bt* toxin resistance in transgenic crops.

TABLE 9.5 *Bt* Strains Registered Under Insecticide Act in India

Bt Subspecies	Strain/Serotype	Formulation Type
Bt kurstaki	i. Strain A-97, serotype H-3a	35 WP
	ii. Strain HD-1, serotype 3a, 3b	3.5% ES
Bt israelensis	i. Strain 164, serotype H-14	WP
	ii. Serotype H-14	5% WP
Bt galleriae	Strain R 1593 M, serotype 3a	1.3% FC

9.3 ENTOMOPATHOGENIC FUNGI (EPF)

Entomopathogenic fungi (EPF) play a pivotal role in the biocontrol management of insect pests worldwide. EPF are unicellular, eukaryotic, filamentous fungi that are able to reproduce both sexually and asexually and produce targeted infective propagules (Bahadur, 2018). According to Sung et al. (2008), *Entomophthorales*, *Hypocreales*, and *Neozygitales* orders belong to the majority of EPF. *Verticillium*, *Metarhizium*, *Nomuraea*, *Beauveria*, *Neozygites,* and *Entomophthora* are among the EPF included in most taxonomic groups (Deshpande, 1999). Lepidoptera, Hemiptera, Coleoptera, Orthoptera, Diptera, and Hymenoptera are insect orders which are attacked by EPF. Hypocreales family fungus attacks almost all victims, while *Entomophthorales* infect only a single type of insect pest. They infect mite species, *lepidopterous larvae*, *aphids*, and *thrips* insects (Roberts and Humber, 1981). During pathogenicity of *Beauveria bassiana* (Hypocreales: Cordycipitaceae) against whitefly of sweet potato (*Bemisia tabaci* G.) after sowing on different host plants viz., cucumber, green pepper, tomato, melon, potato, marrow, eggplant, bean, cabbage, and cotton host plants revealed a strong pathogenicity of *B. bassiana* to the *B. tabaci.* Host plants also influenced the mortality of nymphs caused by *B. bassiana,* whereas newly formed conidia were affected by the host plant. The use of EPF in the management of insect pests is an effective and most desirable approach which involves the utilization of entomopathogenic microorganisms which act as an alternative to chemical pesticides. EPF genera like *Metarhizium, Beauveria, Isaria, Lecanicillium,* and *Hirsutella* act as pesticides in greenhouses, storage facilities, agricultural settings, and residential areas (Sharma and Sharma, 2021). *Beauveria* and *Lecanicillium* kill the insects and are found effective against plant diseases (Kim et al., 2008). Antibiosis and induced resistance mechanisms may be used by *Beauveria* (Benhamou and Brodeur, 2001). EPFs are the most important biological control agent against a variety of insect pests and are cost-effective and eco-friendly (Wraight et al., 2001). EPF have certain characters which help as a component in the IPM program. Commercially available EPF (Butt et al., 2001; De Faria and Wraight, 2007; Kachhawa, 2017; Milner, 2000; Mishra et al., 2015) are listed in Table 9.6.

TABLE 9.6 Commercially Available EPF

EPF	Brand Name	Target Pest	Country
Beauveria bassiana	Mycotrol WP	Whiteflies; aphids; thrips	USA
	Myco-Jaal	Diamondback moth	India
Metarhizium anisopliae	Metaquino	Spittle bugs	Brazil
	DeepGreen	White grub	Colombia
M. anisopliae var. acridum	Green Muscle	Locusts; grasshoppers	South Africa
	Green Muscle	Locusts	China
Nomuraea rileyi	Numoraea 50	Lepidoptera	Colombia
Hirsutella thompsonii	Mycohit	Acari	India
B. bassiana + M. anisopliae + I. fumosoroseus	Tri-Sin	Psyllid	Mexico

9.3.1 MODE OF INFECTION OF EPF ON TARGETED INSECTS

Most EPF are soil borne in nature and have a similar mode of infection on targeted pests. When conidia of fungus come in contact with the host, they immediately attach to the pest cuticle through hydrophobic mechanisms and initiate germ tubes in favorable environmental conditions (Inglis et al., 2001). After attachment, EPF produces various infection structures (penetration pegs, appressoria) which help hyphae to penetrate mycelium into host integument (Ortiz-Urquiza and Keyhani, 2013). Various enzymes like metalloid proteases and amino peptidases are involved during germ tube penetration into pest cuticle (Bidochka and Small, 2005). After penetration of germ tubes, fungi grow as hyphal bodies and disseminate through haemocoel and invade mitochondria, fatty bodies, diverse muscle tissues, Malpighian tubes, and hemocytes, causing death within 5–14 days (Kachhawa, 2017). EPF usually cause insect mortality by release of toxins, destruction of tissues, and by nutritional deficiency. Chitinase, protease, and lipase enzymes secreted from EPF catalyze insect cuticle, and fungal germ tubes penetrate and break down cuticle, further disseminating into the insect body. The entry of EPF germ tubes and fungal infection occur due to mechanical pressure and enzymatic degradation. *B. bassiana*, *V. lecanii*, *Paecilomyces* spp., *M. anisopliae* (Beauvericin, Bassianolide Beauverolides and Destruxins A, B, C, D, E, F), produce several mycotoxins during pathogenesis process which act like poison to the targeted insects. Aerial mycelium of EPF fungus emerges from integument and produce conidial spores on dead insect body.

Entomopthorales group fungi are obligate in nature on insects and kill host by tissue degradations (Pell, 2001).

9.3.2 MASS PRODUCTION

In the laboratory, EPF is maintained on Potato Dextrose Agar Media (Potato 200 gm, dextrose 40 gm, agar 20 gm, yeast 2–5 gm, and distilled water 1000 ml) and sabouraud dextrose agar (dextrose 40 gm, peptone 10 gm, agar 20 gm, yeast 2–5 gm, distilled water 1000 ml, and pH 6.0–6.5) media. For mass multiplication of EPF, sorghum grains are soaked overnight for 24 hours in distilled water. After decanting the water, soaked grains are transferred into a conical flask @ 200 gm/500 ml of flask and autoclaved. All grain-filled flasks are autoclaved at 15 lbs/psi for 15 minutes. Flasks are carefully taken out from the autoclave and kept in the laminar flow chamber for inoculation of EPF. A 10-day-old culture of EPF grown on PDA is cut with the help of a cork borer in the size of a 5mm disk, transferred to SDA-containing Petri plates, and kept for growth in a BOD incubator at 28°C. This freshly grown culture of EPF is cut with a cork borer and aseptically transferred into a conical flask. These conical flasks are incubated at 28°C for 3–4 weeks. After 18–20 days, the sorghum grain gets colonized, covered by the whitish chalky or fluffy growth of EPF. When the grain is fully covered with EPF growth, the colonized grain is dried at 40°C for 96 hours, and the dry grains covered with EPF mycelium are ground into powder form with the help of a mixture grinder. The spore-forming units per gram of powder are counted, and accordingly, $CaCO_3$ additives, sawdust, soybean flour, and ashes are added to make the product. The minimum colony-forming unit (CFU) in additives must be 1 x 106 spores/gm for the long life of spores. Talc ($CaCO_3$) is a very good additive for the storage of EPF for a long duration. The viability of talc-based EPF formulation spores reduced by 27% when stored for 150 days, but at 90 days, the reduction is about 13%. When EPF is used in field conditions, a sticker/spreader must be added before spraying EPF to get optimum results. The sticker/spreader helps in sticking EPF spores properly on the insect cuticle. Most of the time, Tween 20 or a solution of gur is used as a sticker, and washing soap or washing powder is used as a spreader in the field. Around 1 kg of EPF powder in 200 liters of water/acre gave excellent results under field conditions.

9.3.3 APPLICATION

For application of EPF, dissolve 750 gm of biopower/acre along with conventional insecticides/synthetic pyrethroids or 1000 gm/acre to be applied along with the wetting agent in 200 liters of water and apply preferably in the morning or evening.

- **Soil Drenching:** Dissolve 1800 gm of bio-power in 400 liters of water and drench the soil thoroughly for control of root grubs.

9.3.3.1 BIOTECHNOLOGICAL APPLICATION OF EPF

Various mycoacaricides and mycoinsecticides developed worldwide are based on *Beauveria* (33.9%), *B. brongniartii* (4.1%), *Isaria* (5.8%), and *Metarhizium* (33.9%) (deFaria and Wraight, 2007; Sandhu et al., 2012). Recently, research has focused on the production of hyphomycete genera *Metarhizium, Beauveria, Verticillium*, and *Paecilomyces*, which are highly species-specific and have a broad host range (Kaur et al., 2010; Sandhu et al., 2012). Commercial products based on *B. bassiana* are relatively most effective and more stable against lepidopteran insect pests compared to other biological control agents (Rana et al., 2008; Thakur et al., 2011). Selection of high virulent strains requires continued selection of strains with the most stable, highly specific, and efficacious traits for a target host; this was limited by the high degree of genetic diversity (Neves and Hirose, 2005). Wild-type strains are improved by combining different strains and mutant characteristics (Kaur et al., 2010). The efficacy and host range of bioinsecticides will be enhanced through genetic improvement. Molecular biology provides desirable tools for identifying the various mechanisms of pathogenesis and, in the longer run, for producing recombinant organisms with fresh and relevant features. Desired exploration for *M. anisopliae* and *B. bassiana* occurred (Fang et al., 2009). A few necessary genetic transformation systems have been established for manipulation of virulent genes under *in vitro* and *in vivo* conditions (Hasan et al., 2002; Sandhu and Vikrant, 2006). To isolate specific pathogenic genes, transformation techniques have been used to investigate these virulence genes of *Metarhizium* and *Beauveria*, and produced a strain with enhanced virulence. Genetic engineering of EPF will provide a basis for biotechnological mechanisms of fungal pathogenesis in insects. Using cDNA libraries, EST analysis of *B. bassiana* has been studied (Cho et al., 2006). Distinct patterns of proteases and pathogenicity of two subspecies of *M. anisopliae* were revealed through EST analysis. These expression patterns helped the ability to examine gene expression during insect host infection (Freimoser et al., 2005). In this context, much importance has been given to chitinase and proteinase enzymes (Fang et al., 2005) and the metabolic mechanism for the production of insect-specific fungal toxins such as *beauvericin*, *bassianolide*, *isarolides*, and *beauverolides* from *B. bassiana*, and *destruxins* (DTXs) and cytochalasins from *M. anisopliae* (Lozano-Gutiérrez and España-Luna, 2008). Similarly, the virulence of pathogen *B. bassiana* against *Myzus persicae* was enhanced by the release of protein with combined protease and chitinase activities (Fang et al., 2009).

9.3.3.2 BENEFITS OF EPF

- It is an environmentally friendly bio-control agent.
- It is residue-free.
- It controls insect pests that are not possibly controlled by chemical pesticides.
- It is cheaper than pesticides.
- It minimizes losses and the cost of production and increases yield and profit.

9.4 ENTOMOPATHOGENIC NEMATODES (EPN)

Nematodes are among the most abundant groups of living animals. Morphologically, they are simple and exploited in diverse habitats, including invertebrates. They are considered pests to humans and animals, as well as agricultural crops, and are responsible for economic loss of produce. EPNs are considered potential biocontrol agents of pests, as they are associated with insects, *spiders*, *annelids*, *leeches*, *crustaceans*, and *molluscs*. A total of nine families of nematodes (Allantonematidae, Diplogasteridae, Heterorhabditidae, Mermithidae, Neotylechidae, Rhabditidae, Sphaerulariidae, Steinernematidae, and Tetradonematidae) are able to kill insects and also alter their development. *Photorhabdus* and *Xenorhabdus* bacterial genera show a mutualistic relationship with *Heterorhabditis* and *Steinernema* group nematodes, respectively, and are also pathogenic to host insects (Ferreira and Malan, 2014). The insecticidal potential of these nematodes has been examined against various insect species, including lepidopteran pests around the world (Begley, 1990; Grewal et al., 2005; Hussain and Ahmad, 2011; Lacey and Georgis, 2012). Under favorable conditions, EPNs are lethal parasites, and infective juvenile nematodes search for insect larvae and pupae in the soil. EPNs penetrate natural body openings of the insect (mouth, anus, and spiracles), and the bacteria released kill the insects within a day. Killed insects become flaccid and have conspicuous colors. Insects killed by *Steinernema carpocapsae* turn yellow in color, while *Heterorhabditis bacteriophora* are reddish brown. After the death of the insect, nematodes feed on bacteria as well as the body contents of the host and reproduce. Within a week, infective juveniles are released into the soil to search out new hosts and continue their life cycle. EPNs against target pests are listed in Table 9.7.

TABLE 9.7 Use of EPN Against Insects

Crop	EPN	Target Insect
Cabbage	*S. carpocapsae, H. bacteriophora*	*Plutella xylostella*
Rice	*S. carpocapsae*	*Tryporyza incertudus*
Sugarcane	*S. carpocapsae*	*Tryporyza incertudus*
Maize	*S. riobave*	*Helicoverpa armigera*
	S. feltiae	*Diabrotica barberi*
Cotton	*S. carpocapsae*	*Spodoptera littoralis, E. insulana*
Potato	*S. carpocapsae*	*Anomala* spp., *Earias insulana*
Brinjal	*S. carpocapsae, H. indica*	*Leucinodes orbonalis*
Pigeon pea	*H. indica*	*Helicoverpa armigera*
Citrus	*S. carpocapsae*	*Phyllocnistis citrella*
		Diaprepes abbreviatus

9.4.1 LIFE CYCLE AND HOST RANGE OF STEINERNEMATIDAE AND HETERORHABDITIDAE EPNS

The life cycle of EPNs includes the eggs, four juvenile stages, and the adults. The infective stage is the third-stage juvenile, which is resistant to the environmental conditions. Infective-stage juveniles (IJs) are ensheathed with an intact J2 cuticle. This extra cuticle provides resistance to the environmental conditions for the juvenile. The IJs are the only free-living forms occurring outside the host. They do not feed and can survive long periods in soil in favorable conditions. The life cycles of both species (*Steinernematids* and *Heterorhabditids*) are similar, except that *Heterorhabditids* can enter either through natural openings or even actively puncture the cuticle and directly reach the hemocoel with the help of a tooth. The IJs then develop into hermaphroditic females. These females produce a sexual generation that reproduces to form a new set of hermaphroditic infective juveniles.

Steinernematids and *Heterorhabditids* have been observed to infect more than 200 species of insects from several orders. Some of the insects controlled are armyworm, carpenter worm, cat fleas, crown borers, cutworms, filth flies, flea beetles, leaf miner, phorid flies, plum moths, root weevils, stem borer, webworm, and white grubs (Kleint, 1990). Commercially available EPNs are listed in Table 9.8 (Dunn, 1997).

TABLE 9.8 Commercial EPN

EPN Species	Product Formulation	Country
Steinernema carpocapsae	Green commandos, soil commandos	India
S. carpocapsae	Bio vector	USA
	Exhibit	USA
	Ortho biosafe	USA
S. feltiae	Nemasys	UK
	Stealth	UK
S. riobave	Bio vector	USA
Heterorhabditis bacteriophora	Otinem	USA
Heterorhabditis megidis	Nemasys	UK

9.4.2 *MASS PRODUCTION AND STORAGE OF EPN*

EPNs have been cultured on a variety of substrates such as ground veal pulp, potato mash, homogenized animal tissues, peptone–glucose agar, and pork kidney, chicken offal, and dog food, and so forth. EPNs infect and reproduce on insects and can also be reared *in vivo* in the laboratory. *Galleria mellonella* is the most preferred host used worldwide because of its ease of rearing, high susceptibility, and suitability for nematode reproduction. However, other hosts like *S. litura, Corcyra cephalonica, Chilo sacchariphagus indicus, Scirpophaga excerptalis,* and *Bombyx mori* may also be used for rearing purposes. A population of 465,000 IJs of *S. abbasi* and up to 535,000 of *H. indica* have been harvested from a single larva of *G. mellonella* under *in vivo* conditions.

For mass production on *G. mellonella*, the IJs suspension should be warmed to room temperature (20–24°C), then dilute 1.0 ml of sterile water to yield approximately 200 nematodes/ml. Count the IJs and adjust the suspension to 200 nematodes/ml. Distribute 1.0 ml of nematode suspension on 9.0 cm Whatman filter paper in the lid of a (100 × 14 cm) plastic Petri plate. Add *Galleria* larvae and cover the lid with the inverted Petri plate bottom. All Petri plates should be carefully stored at ambient temperature, and then infected larvae placed into white traps for 5–7 days after infection. Harvesting is done by placing a 9.0 cm Whatman filter paper in a concave side up watch glass in a large glass Petri plate. Place infected larvae (10–25 as they fit) on the filter paper over the edge of the watch glass. IJs will start to exit 10–12 days after infection. For harvesting, remove the watch glass with dead larvae, pour the IJs into a beaker, add 70 ml of SDW or 0.1% formalin, and replace the watch glass. Allow the rinsed IJs to settle in a beaker, then centrifuge at 300 rpm for 1 minute to speed settling and transfer the nematodes into a storage container.

9.4.3 APPLICATION OF EPN

EPNs can be sprayed by using various sprayers and irrigation systems (Shapiro-Ilan et al., 2015). EPNs can be delivered in combination with other biocontrol agents, synthetic insecticides, plant growth-promoting rhizobacteria (PGPR), and fertilizer. They can be applied with an irrigation system.

1. **Combined Application with Other Biocontrol Agents:** Combined application of two EPN species against *A. ipsilon* larvae and *Listronotus maculicollis* (Koppenhöfer et al., 2015) has been responsible for the mortality. Combined application of *Bacillus* (*Btj*) and EPNs did not have synergistic effects on white grub (Koppenhöfer et al., 1999). Both *H. megidis* and *S. glaseri* revealed a strong synergistic interaction with *M. anisopliae* in second and third-instar *Hoplia philanthus* when applied 34 weeks before the EPNs (Ansari et al., 2006).
2. **Combined Application with Insecticides:** The combination of Imidacloprid and *H. bacteriophora* yielded the most consistent synergism against third instar white grubs, but a high rate of control was observed against second and third instars grubs using

minimum rates of 25% and a full rate of 50% for *H. bacteriophora* and imidacloprid (Koppenhöfer and Fuzy, 2008).

3. **Combined Application with Beneficial Microorganisms:** Application of *H. bacteriophora, S. feltiae, H. megidis* and combined with *Pseudomonas* spp. and arbuscular mycorrhizal fungi to wheat (Imperiali et al., 2017) and corn (Jaffuel et al., 2019) also gave a positive response.
4. **Soil Application:** Spraying EPN on the soil surface is the best method for EPN application. One billion nematodes per acre is the recommended rate for the broadcast application of EPNs to control most soil insects (Vashisth et al., 2013). The soil should be well irrigated, and the soil temperature should be in the range of 12 to 28°C for the survival and movement of EPNs. If the temperature is more than 28°C, then pre-irrigation should be applied before EPN application. Nematode mobility is always greater in sandy soil as compared to clay soil.
5. **Foliar Application:** EPNs are mostly applied on standing crops by spray. Nozzle type, spraying procedure, and spray droplet size influence the EPN spray and deposition on plant leaves. However, additives always increased the deposition of nematodes on leaves, while tinpal, ujal, and ranipal decrease the high temperature and UV radiation that indirectly save the EPNs.
6. **Trickle Application of EPN:** A button type of trickle irrigation outlet is used to deliver the inoculums to the area on one side of the plant.
7. **Capsules Application of EPN:** Recently, the EPN has been used in the form of a capsule, which is very suitable under soil conditions. Wheat bran (5%) with calcium alginate is mostly used for making EPN capsules. One capsule contains 1000–2000 nematodes. About 70–80 capsules/plant could be enough for application.

9.4.4 *CHARACTERS OF EPN*

- It has a high searching capacity for target insects in soil and on plant surfaces.

- It is able to kill the target insect quickly by releasing bacteria into the host body.
- It has a broad host range, including Lepidoptera, Coleoptera, Orthoptera, Diptera, Homoptera, and others.
- It can be easily recovered from soil and multiplied within a short period of time.
- It is easily culturable using an artificial diet as well as on living host insects.
- EPNs are very much compatible with a broad range of pesticides, and they can be formulated as dust, sprays, capsules, granules, and so forth, and applied as an EPN suspension through spraying and irrigation systems.
- EPNs are safe for plants, vertebrates, and non-target organisms.
- EPNs are safe for the environment and eco-friendly in nature.
- No registration is required for mass multiplication.

9.4.5 BIOTECHNOLOGICAL APPLICATION IN EPN

Due to environmental extremes and their host-finding behavior, EPNs are susceptible in field situations. To improve their efficacy, artificial selection, hybridization, mutagenesis, and recombinant DNA technology can be used (Dhaliwal et al., 2013). Genetically engineered EPNs have been improved by the development of recent advances in molecular biology techniques. Hashmi et al. (1995) was the first to successfully transform *Heterorhabditis bacteriophora* HP88 by microinjection of plasmid vectors. The first cDNA-sequencing project of the EPNs was ESTs generated in *H. bacteriophora* strain GPS11; 1072 ESTs were categorized into functional categories, and 613 ESTs did not match in any of the searched databases, suggesting potentially novel genes in the EPNs. About 81 unique ESTs were identified in the IS-6 strain of *Steinernema feltiae* on desiccation (Gal et al., 2003). Out of these, genes Sf-ALDH, Hsp40, ubq-2, and glycerol kinase were upregulated only during 8 to 24 h of desiccation; however, Sf-LEA-1 of LEA (late embryogenesis abundant) was highly upregulated even after 24 h of desiccation. Hao et al. (2010) observed cDNA transcripts expressed in *S. carpocapsae* to find genes involved in parasitism. About 32% of the total ESTs generated had no homology with any known gene in public databases, which showed the presence of novel genes involved in the parasitism of EPN. Ciche and Sternberg (2007) have already indicated the feasibility of postembryonic RNAi in *H. bacteriophora* through soaking, which may be a potent approach for studying gene-function in EPNs. The immune response of *H. parallela* against EPNs infection achieved and validated three crucial immune-related RNAi genes technology (Ertao, 2021). These genomic resources may be able to generate genetically modified *H. bacteriophora*. These approaches may be extended to develop more genetically improved strains of the other EPN species.

9.5 ENTOMOPATHOGENIC VIRUS

Entomopathogenic viruses have a pivotal role in controlling different crop pests. They are submicroscopic and obligate intracellular pathogenic entities belonging to 11 families (Fauquet et al. 2004), including Baculoviridae, Reoviridae, Iridoviridae, Poxviridae, Parvoviridae, Picornaviridae, Rhabdoviridae, and others. Out of this limited group of insect viruses, viruses belonging to Baculoviridae act as the prominent player due to their specificity, pathogenicity, environmental persistence, narrow host range, and compatibility with other bio-agents. Besides, they have less toxic residual effects and pest resistance compared to conventional pesticides (Barreto et al., 2005; Zhang et al., 2005).

9.5.1 THE BACULOVIRUSES CLASSIFICATION AND HOST RANGE

Baculoviruses are double-stranded DNA (dsDNA) viruses and are identified based on inclusion bodies (IBs). The virions of the *Baculoviridae* are a rod-shaped virus family and have a virion particle size of 40–70 nm X 250–400 nm, comprising an envelope of lipoprotein around the protein capsid, which contains a DNA-protein core. Baculoviruses have large, circular, and dsDNA genomes (81.7 to 178.7 kb) (Zhang et al., 2005).

The Baculoviridae family comprises the subfamilies Eubaculovirinae and Nudibaculovirinae, in which virions are encapsulated within a crystalline protein matrix (Francki et al., 1991). Eubaculovirinae includes the genera Nuclear Polyhedrosis Virus (NPV) and Granulosis Virus (GV), which can be differentiated based on their shape, size, and virion phenotype. GV capsules contain small occlusion bodies (OBs) (0.25–0.5 μm in cross section), whereas NPV polyhedra contain large OBs (0.15–15 μm) (Braunagel et al., 2003).

The baculoviruses infect only Lepidoptera, Coleoptera, Diptera, Hymenoptera, Neuroptera, Trichoptera, Mites, and Crustacea and do not multiply in plants and microorganisms. NPV has been exploited commercially and registered worldwide under different trade names across the globe, and it has particularly been successful in managing two major polyphagous pests such as *H. armigera* and *S. litura.*

9.5.2 NUCLEAR POLYHEDROSIS VIRUS (NPV)

NPV is a naturally occurring, self-perpetuating virus which is safe to natural enemies due to its host specificity. The polyhedral capsid of the virus is a stable protein crystal that protects the virus from other environmental factors. NPV dissolves in the midgut of moths and butterflies, which contain alkaline pH, and releases infective virus particles, affecting the larva (Chiu et al., 2012).

1. **Structure:** During the infection, NPV produces virions like Budded Virion (BV) and Occluded body derived virions (ODV) having identical genotypes, but distinct phenotypes. In addition, they possess similar nucleocapsids differing only in their envelopes. The envelopes of BVs are resultant of modified plasma membranes, while the envelopes of Occluded bodies are resultant of membranes assembled within the nucleus (Ikeda et al., 2015). Baculoviruses have only a single nucleocapsid envelope, whereas ODVs embedded within ocular bodies consist of either single or multiple nucleocapsids and are referred to as SNPVs or MNPVs. OBs are required for virus survival and transmission.
2. **Infection and Appearance of Symptom:** Larvae ingest contaminated food with occluded bodies (OBs), having infectious ODVs. The ingested OBs get dissolved in the alkaline digestive juice of the insect midgut lumen and release ODVs, which adsorb on microvilli of midgut columnar cells. The ODV envelopes plasma membranes help nucleocapsids to penetrate into the cytoplasm. Then nucleocapsids move into the nucleus by actin-based motility (Ohkawa et al., 2010), where the capsid is uncoated and releases the DNA. Afterwards, genomic DNA replicates and expresses late genes to produce structural proteins within the infected nucleus (Nagamine et al., 2011) and form new replicates of viruses after morphogenesis of nucleocapsids. Newly formed viruses enter the cytoplasm of midgut epithelial cells and bud from plasma

membranes modified by baculovirus-encoded envelope fusion proteins to form enveloped BVs. BVs enter into the haemocoel of the insect using tracheal cells as a conduit (Passarelli, 2011). Nucleocapsids are enveloped within the nucleus to form ODVs, which are embedded within OBs and remain in the nucleus and released into the environment after the death of larvae by liquefaction. Therefore, ODVs embedded in OBs transmit horizontally from insects to insects, whereas BVs transfer cell-to-cell within the insect body.

Unlike ODVs, BVs enter through adsorptive endocytosis (Katou et al., 2010) where proteins GP64 and F-proteins bind to plasma membrane receptors of the host. Then, the viral membrane and the cell plasma membrane are fused, creating a low pH that triggers the membrane penetration of the nucleocapsid. After binding to the cell surface, BVs migrate to the nucleus and trigger membrane fusion between the BV envelope and endosomal membrane, permitting the release of nucleocapsids into the cytoplasm. Then, nucleocapsids are uncoated to release the viral particle and start replication.

Infected larvae hang upside down, and their integument changes in color, later becoming flaccid and fragile. Besides, larvae become sluggish, wet, and experience discoloration of skin, and regurgitation of fluids. The larvae become swollen, turn black with decay, and contain virions of the virus after death (Figures 9.1 and 9.2). After death, the body wall of the larvae ruptures, and OBs are released.

3. **Commercial Product of NPV: World and India:** Various NPV-based pesticides are registered in different countries under different names. Elcar™ was one of the first such viral insecticides announced by Sandoz in 1975 (Ignoffo and Couch, 1981). *Heliothis zea* NPV (Elcar™), a broad-range baculovirus, infects many species of *Helicoverpa* and *Heliothis* (Chakraborty et al., 1999). *Neodiprion sertifer* NPV has been successfully applied for control of the European pine sawfly, which is a serious pest on pine plantations (Cunningham and Entwistle, 1981), and commercial products were registered in Finland (1983), UK (1985), and USA (1983). *Autographa californica* MNPV has a broad host range

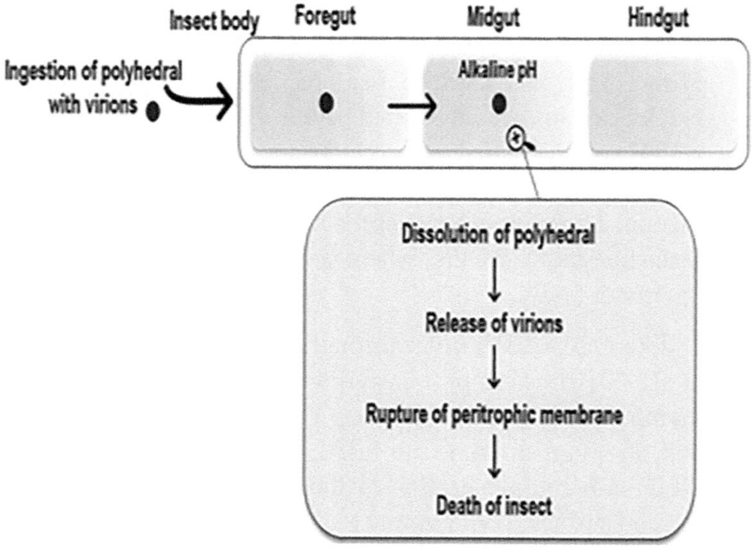

FIGURE 9.1 Infection process.

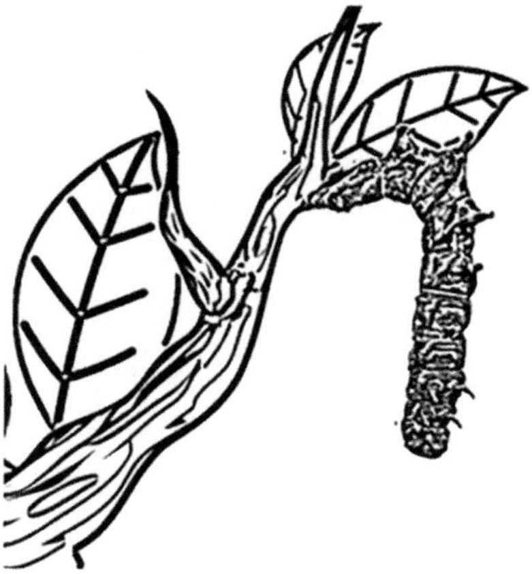

FIGURE 9.2 Symptom.

and has been tested for control of different insects, especially of *Heliothis virescens* and *Trichoplusia ni*. AcMNPV has been registered in the USA since 1994. Experimental and commercial use of AcMNPV is reported from Central America (Guatemala), where it has been applied on several thousand hectares of cabbage and broccoli (Hunter-Fujita and Frances, 1998). *Spodoptera* NPVs are currently in use in the USA, and another in Europe in the name of SPOD-X™, containing *Spodoptera exigua* NPV for controlling insects on vegetable crops, and Spodopterin™, containing *Spodoptera littoralis* NPV in cotton, corn, and tomatoes (Szewczyket al., 2006). Likewise, NPVs of *S. littoralis* and *S. exempta* in Egypt and Kenya, and *Anticarsia gemmatalis* NPV are used in different trade names in Brazil. China used 12 Baculovirus-based insecticides (Sun and Peng, 2007), including *H. armigera* NPV (cotton, pepper, and tobacco), *S. litura* NPV and *S. exigua* NPV (vegetables), and *Buzura suppressaria* NPV (tea). The NPV-based, well-known bio-pesticide *Anticarsia gemmatalis* nucleopolyhedrovirus (AgMNPV) is used against the velvet bean caterpillar of soybean (Moscardi, 1999) in 2,000,000 ha. In temperate forests, defoliators like *Lymantria dispar, Orgyia pseudotsugata, Lymantria monacha,* and *Panolis flammea* are controlled by *L. dispar* MNPV, which was available in trade names of Gypchek and Virin-ENSH, and *O. pseudotsugata* MNPV (BioControl-1 and Virtuss) (Reardon et al., 1996) has been used in the USA in forest ecosystems.

Among the NPVs, only *H. armigera* (HaNPV) and *S. litura* (SlNPV) have been exploited on tomato, cotton, groundnut, chickpea, and field bean (Srinivasa et al., 2008). Spodo-Cide®, Spodopterin®, Heli-Cide®, Heliokill®, and so forth, are biopesticides marketed under different trade names in India (Ramanujam et al., 2014). Commercial formulations of NPV are listed in Table 9.9.

4. **Mass Production of NPV:** Since NPV is an obligate parasite, it multiplies only in living larvae. So, mass production of NPV is a tedious job and requires skilled labor (McIntosh et al., 1987). Mass production of NPV is the same for *S. litura* and *H. armigera*, but in the case of *H. armigera*, it can be reared in separate vials to avoid cannibalism. Both natural as well as artificial diets can be used for mass production of NPV contaminated with the respective pests. The field-collected or laboratory-reared third instar larvae of both the pests are allowed to feed on the NPV-contaminated diet. The larvae are reared in 5 mL glass vials containing diet until they reach the appropriate developmental stage and are then used for production. The 10 mL aliquots of viral suspension (POB, 1 × 108) are spread uniformly over the center of the diet. After 15

min, larvae are released singly into each glass vial and incubated at 25°C for 10 days. From the fifth day onwards, larvae start to die. The dead larvae are collected and transferred to containers and frozen. The infected larvae are crushed in a mixer cum grinder by adding sufficient water. Then, the solution is repeatedly filtered using muslin cloth. Afterwards, the solution may be centrifuged (30,000 RPM) to separate the polyhedral body of NPV, and this will be separated from water for further use (Sridhar et al., 2008). PIB can be counted under a dark field or phase-contrast microscope using a hemocytometer. The dose of virus is passed as larval equivalent (LE), and one LE is 6 x 109 POB. Three NPV-infected fully grown larvae are required to produce one LE.

5. **Method of Application**: NPV can be applied in the field late in the evening after peak sunshine hours for getting the most effective results. NPV is highly susceptible to ultraviolet light (sunlight) and high-temperature conditions, but it will survive years together in a protected environment. Hence, the use of 1 ml of robin blue nil (UV absorbents) in 1 liter of solution is recommended for the enhancement of NPV action. For chickpea, pigeonpea, and cotton, HaNPV should be used @ 250–300 LE, 500 LE, and 250 LE/ha, respectively.

TABLE 9.9 Commercial Formulations of NPV

Name of NPV	Trade Name of the Product	Country
Heliothis zea NPV	Elcar™	USA
Neodiprion sertifer NPV	Neochek-S	USA
Neodiprion lecontei NPV	Lecontvirus®	USA and Canada
Spodoptera exigua NPV	SPOD-X™	USA and Europe
Spodoptera littoralis NPV	Spodopterin™	USA and Europe
Lymantria dispar NPV	Gypchek, Disparivirus, Virin-ENSH	USA
Orgyia pseudotsugata NPV	BioControl-1 and Virtuss	USA
Helicoverpa armigera NPV	Heli-Cide®, Heliokill®	India
Spodoptera litura NPV	Spodo-Cide®, Spodopterin®	India
Mamestra brassicae	Mamestrin	France
Anticarsia gemmatalis NPV	Baculo-soja Coopervirus SC	Brazil
Autographa californica NPV + *Spodoptera albula* NPV	VPN-ULTRA	Guatemala

9.5.3 *BIOTECHNOLOGICAL APPLICATION FOR EFFECTIVENESS OF NPV*

Due to its slow speed of insect mortality, widespread dissemination and use of NPV has never been achieved. The use of genetic engineering can offer scope to NPVs to kill insects more efficiently in a shorter time (Guo et al., 2006). The baculovirus is used for genetic engineering for cloning various insecticidal proteins like PTTH, toxins, *trehalase*, juvenile hormone esterase, melittin, scorpion and mite toxins, and fungal insecticidal protease into NPV (Charmi et al., 2009). In this regard, some of the genes having faster killing properties have been inserted through genetic engineering (Table 9.10), and further research is in progress.

TABLE 9.10 Development of Genetically Engineered NPVs

NPV	Foreign Gene	Host Insect	References
BmNPV	AaIT Toxin from *Andractomus australis*	*Bombyx mori*	Inceoglu et al. (2001)
AcMNPV	Toxin 21 A, from *Pyemotes tritici*	*Trichoplusia ni*	Burden et al. (2000)
AcMNPV and HvJHE	BmK IT, Neurotoxin from Spider	*S. exigua*	Fan et al. (2008)

9.6 CONCLUSION AND FUTURE THRUST

Microbial pathogens (bacteria, fungi, nematode, and virus) have long been recognized as one of the potential biopesticides, as they are easy to handle, have less residual toxicity, are eco-friendly and compatible with other synthetic chemical pesticides, and are self-perpetuating in nature. The development of resistance to chemical pesticides has also secured the development of entomopathogens, and they can be used as an integral part of an IPM component. Besides, for the past 25 years, the investigation tactic on insect pathogens has changed toward being more ecologically feasible with industry's concerns but is still facing many constraints in production, marketing, and use. Hence, to make it more successful commercially, quality control guidelines and methodologies need to be developed. There should be a strong and systematic registration policy to find out more virulent and ultraviolet-resistant strains. For commercial success of the product, development of an *in vitro* production system is very much essential. There is a great scope of utilizing genetically modified entomopathogens that will progressively occupy space in the pesticide industry. Hence, there is a dire need for effective multidisciplinary research and public-private-people partnerships to arise with entomopathogens that can spread in wider environments, effectively covering a large host range.

KEYWORDS

- **baculovirus**
- **entomopathogens**
- **genetic engineering**
- ***in vitro* production system**
- **microbial pathogens**
- **pesticides**
- **ultraviolet**

REFERENCES

Adams, J. R., & McClintock, J. T. (1991). Nuclear polyhedrosis viruses of insects. In J. R. Adams & J. R. Bonami (Eds.), *Atlas of Invertebrate Viruses* (pp. 87–204). CRC Press.

Andreeva, I. V., & Chternchis, M. V. (1995). Microbiologitcheskie preparati protif pautinovo klesha v tiplitsah. *Zashita Rastenii, 11*, 41–42.

Ansari, M. A., Shah, F. A., Tirry, L., & Moens, M. (2006). Field trials against *Hoplia philanthus* (Coleoptera: Scarabaeidae) with a combination of an entomopathogenic nematode and the fungus *Metarhizium anisopliae* CLO 53. *Biological Control, 39*, 453–459.

Bahadur, A. (2018). Entomopathogens: Role of insect pest management in crops. *Trends in Horticulture, 1*, 1–9. https://doi.org/10.24294/th.v1i4.833 (accessed on 2nd January 2026).

Barreto, M. R., Guimaraes, C. T., Teixeira, F. F., Paiva, E., & Valicente, F. H. (2005). Effect of *Baculovirus spodoptera* isolates in *Spodoptera frugiperda* (J.E. Smith) (Lepidoptera: Noctuidae) larvae and their characterization by RAPD. *Neotropical Entomology, 34*(1), 67–75.

Begley, J. W. (1990). Efficacy against insects in habitats other than soil. In R. Gaugler & H. K. Kaya (Eds.), *Entomopathogenic Nematodes in Biological Control* (pp. 215–231). CRC Press.

Benhamou, N., & Brodeur, J. (2001). Pre-inoculation of Ri T-DNA transformed cucumber roots with the mycoparasite, *Verticillium lecanii*, induces host defense reactions against *Pythium ultimum* infection. *Physiological and Molecular Plant Pathology, 58*, 133–146.

Bidochka, M. J., & Small, C. (2005). Phylogeography of *Metarhizium*, an insect pathogenic fungus. In F. E. Vega & M. Blackwell (Eds.), *Insect-Fungal Associations* (pp. 28–49). Oxford University Press.

Braunagel, S. C., Russell, W. K., Rosas Acosta, G., Russell, D. H., & Summers, M. D. (2003). Determination of protein composition of the occlusion-derived virus of *Autographa californica* nucleopolyhedrovirus. *Proceedings of the National Academy of Sciences of the United States of America, 100*, 9797–9802.

Bravo, A., Likitvivatanavong, S., & Gill, S. S. (2011). *Bacillus thuringiensis*: A story of a successful bioinsecticide. *Insect Biochemistry and Molecular Biology, 41*, 423–431.

Burden, J. P., Hails, R. S., Windass, J. D., Suner, M., & Cory, J. S. (2000). Infectivity, speed of kill, and productivity of a baculovirus expressing the Itch Mite Toxin Txp-1 in second and fourth instar larvae of *Trichoplusia ni*. *Journal of Invertebrate Pathology, 75*(3), 226–236.

Butt, T. M., Harris, J. G., & Powell, K. A. (1999). Microbial biopesticides. In F. R. Hall & J. J. Menn (Eds.), *Methods in Biotechnology, 5, Biopesticides: Use and Delivery* (pp. 266–269). Humana Press.

Butt, T. M., Jackson, C. W., & Magan, N. (2001). *Fungal Biological Control Agents: Progress, Problems and Potentials*. CABI International.

Chakraborty, S., Monsour, C., Teakle, R., & Reid, S. (1999). Yield, biological activity, and field performance of a wild-type *Helicoverpa* nucleopolyhedroviral produced in *H. zea* cell cultures. *Journal of Invertebrate Pathology, 73*, 199–205.

Chiu, E., Coulibaly, F., & Metcalf, P. (2012). Insect virus polyhedra, infectious protein crystals that contain virus particles. *Current Opinion in Structural Biology, 22*(2), 234–240.

Cho, E. M., Liu, L., Farmerie, W., & Keyhani, N. O. (2006). EST analysis of cDNA libraries from the entomopathogenic fungus *Beauveria* (*Cordyceps*) *bassiana*. I. Evidence for stage-specific gene expression in aerial conidia, *in vitro* blastospores and submerged conidia. *Microbiology, 152*, 2843–2854.

Ciche, T. A., & Sternberg, P. W. (2007). Postembryonic RNAi in *Heterorhabditis bacteriophora*: A nematode insect parasite and host for insect pathogenic symbionts. *BMC Developmental Biology, 7*, 101.

Cunningham, J. C., & Entwistle, P. F. (1981). Control of sawflies by baculovirus. In H. D. Burges (Ed.), *Microbial Control of Pests and Diseases 1970–1980* (pp. 379–407). Academic Press.

Dara, S. K. (2017). Entomopathogenic microorganisms: Modes of action and role in IPM. *E-Journal of Entomology and Biological*. https://ucanr.edu/blogs/blogcore/postdetail.cfm?postnum=24119 (accessed on 2nd January 2026).

DeFaria, M. R., & Wraight, S. P. (2007). Mycoinsecticides and mycoacaricides: A comprehensive list with worldwide coverage and international classification of formulation types. *Biological Control, 43*, 237–256.

Deshpande, M. V. (1999). Mycopesticide production by fermentation: Potential and challenges. *Critical Reviews in Microbiology, 25*, 229–243.

Dhaliwal, G. S., Singh, R., & Jindal, V. (2013). *A Textbook of Integrated Pest Management* (617 pp.). Kalyani Publishers.

Dunn, P. E. (1997). Biochemical aspects of insect immunity. *Annual Review of Entomology, 31*, 321–339.

Fan, X., Zheng, B., Fu, Y., Sun, Y., & Liang, A. (2008). Baculovirus-mediated expression of a Chinese scorpion neurotoxin improves insecticidal efficacy. *Chinese Science Bulletin, 53*, 1855–1860.

Fang, W. B., Leng, Y., Xia, K., Jin, J. M., Fan, Y., & Feng, J. (2005). Cloning of *Beauveria bassiana* chitinase gene *Bbchit1* and its application to improve fungal strain virulence. *Applied and Environmental Microbiology, 71*, 363–370.

Fang, W., Feng, J., Fan, Y., Zhang, Y., Bidochka, M. J., & St. Leger, R. J. (2009). Expressing a fusion protein with protease and chitinase activities increases the virulence of the insect pathogen *Beauveria bassiana. Journal of Invertebrate Pathology, 102*, 155–159.

Fauquet, C. M., Mayo, M. A., Maniloff, J., Desselberger, U., & Ball, L. A. (2004). *Virus Taxonomy. VII Report of the ICTV* (p. 1258). Elsevier/Academic.

Ferreira, T., & Malan, A. P. (2014). *Xenorhabdus* and *Photorhabdus*, bacterial symbionts of the entomopathogenic nematodes *Steinernema* and *Heterorhabditis* and their *in vitro* liquid mass culture: A review. *African Entomology, 22*, 1–14.

Francki, R. I. B., Fauquet, C. M., Knudson, D., & Brown, F. (1991). Classification and nomenclature of viruses. *Fifth Report of the International Committee on Taxonomy of Viruses. Archives of Virology, Supplement 2.*

Freimoser, M., Hu, G., & St. Leger, R. J. (2005). Variation in gene expression patterns as the insect pathogen *Metarhizium anisopliae* adapts to different host cuticles or nutrient deprivation *in vitro*. *Microbiology, 151*, 361–371.

Gal, T. Z., Glazer, I., & Koltai, H. (2003). Differential gene expression during desiccation stress in the insect-killing nematode *Steinernema feltiae* IS-6. *Journal of Parasitology, 89*, 761–766.

Gill, S. S., Cowles, E. A., & Pietrantonio, P. V. (1992). The mode of action of *Bacillus thuringiensis* endotoxins. *Annual Review of Entomology, 37*, 615–636.

Goettel, M. S., Koike, M., Kim, J. J., Aiuchi, D., Shinya, R., & Brodeur, J. (2008). Potential of *Lecanicillium* spp. for management of insects, nematodes and plant diseases. *Journal of Invertebrate Pathology, 98*(3), 256–261.

Grewal, P. S., Ehlers, R. U., & Shapiro-Ilan, D. I. (2005). *Nematodes as Biocontrol Agents* (p. 505). CABI Publishing.

Guo, Z. J., Ge, J. Q., Wang, D., Shao, Y. M., Tang, Q. Y., & Zang, C. X. (2006). Biological comparison of two genotypes of *Helicoverpa armigera* single-nucleocapsid nucleopolyhedrovirus. *Biological Control.* https://doi.org/10.1007/s1056-006-9008-6 (accessed on 2nd January 2026).

Hao, Y. J., Motiel, R., Abubucker, S., Mitreva, M., & Simoes, N. (2010). Transcript analysis of the entomopathogenic nematodes *Steinernema carpocapsae* induced *in vitro* with insect haemolymph. *Molecular and Biochemical Parasitology, 169*, 79–86.

Hasan, S., Bhamra, A. K., Sil, K., Rajak, R. C., & Sandhu, S. S. (2002). Spore production of *Metarhizium anisopliae* (ENT-12) by solid state fermentation. *Journal of Indian Botanical Society, 8*, 85–88.

Hashmi, S., Hashmi, G., & Gaugler, R. (1995). Genetic transformation of an entomopathogenic nematode by microinjection. *Journal of Invertebrate Pathology, 66*, 293–296.

Hofte, H., & Whitely, H. P. (1989). Insecticidal crystal proteins of *Bacillus thuringiensis. Microbiological and Molecular Biology Reviews, 53*(2), 242–255.

Hunter-Fujita, R. F., Entwistle, P. F., Evans, F. H., & Crook, N. E. (1998). *Insect Virus and Pest Management*. Wiley.

Hussain, M. A., & Ahmad, W. (2011). *Management of Helicoverpa armigera by Entomopathogenic Nematodes* (p. 168). Lambert Academic Publishing GmbH & Co. KG.

Ignoffo, C. M., & Couch, T. L. (1981). The nucleopolyhedrosis virus of *Heliothis* species as a microbial pesticide. In H. Burges (Ed.), *Microbial Control of Pests and Plant Diseases* (pp. 329–362). Academic Press.

Ikeda, M., Hamajima, R., & Kobayashi, M. (2015). Baculoviruses: Diversity, evolution and manipulation of insects. *Entomological Science, 18*, 1–20.

Imperiali, N., Chiriboga, M. X., Schlaeppi, K., Fesselet, M., Villacrés, D., & Jaffuel, G. (2017). Combined field inoculations of *Pseudomonas* bacteria, arbuscular mycorrhizal fungi and entomopathogenic nematodes and their effects on wheat performance. *Frontiers in Plant Science, 8*, 1809. https://doi.org/10.3389/fpls.2017.01809 (accessed on 2nd January 2026).

Inceoglu, A. B., Kamita, S. G., Hinton, A. C., Huang, Q., Severson, T. F., & Kang, K. D. (2001). Recombinant baculoviruses for insect control. *Pest Management Science, 57*, 981–987.

Inglis, G. D., Goettel, M., Butt, T., & Strasser, H. (2001). Use of hyphomycetous fungi for managing insect pests. In T. M. Butt, C. W. Jackson, & N. Magan (Eds.), *Fungi as Biocontrol Agents: Progress, Problems and Potentials* (pp. 23–70). CABI Publishing.

Jaffuel, G., Imperiali, N., Shelby, K., Campos-Herrera, R., Geisert, R., & Maurhofer, M. (2019). Protecting maize from rootworm damage with the combined application of arbuscular mycorrhizal fungi, *Pseudomonas* bacteria and entomopathogenic nematodes. *Scientific Reports, 9*, 1–12. https://doi.org/10.1038/s41598-019-39753-7 (accessed on 2nd January 2026).

James, C. (2016). Global status of commercialized Biotech/GM crops: 2016. *ISAAA Brief No. 52*. http://www.isaaa.org (accessed on 2nd January 2026).

Kachhawa, D. (2017). Microorganisms as a biopesticide. *Journal of Entomology and Zoology Studies, 5*(3), 468–473.

Katou, Y., Yamada, H., Ikeda, M., & Kobayashi, M. (2010). A single amino acid substitution modulates low-pH-triggered membrane fusion of GP64 protein in *Autographa californica* and *Bombyx mori* nucleopolyhedroviruses. *Virology, 404*, 204–214.

Kaur, R., Gupta, V. K., Jindal, V., Blossom, & Dilawari, V. K. (2010). Growing *Beauveria bassiana* for cuticle-degrading activities and its bio-efficacy against greater wax moth *Galleria melonella. Biopesticides International, 6*, 96–104.

Kim, J. J., Goettel, M. S., & Gillespie, D. R. (2008). Evaluation of *Lecanicillium longisporum*, Vertalec for simultaneous suppression of cotton aphid, *Aphis gossypii*, and cucumber powdery mildew, *Sphaerotheca fuliginea*, on potted cucumbers. *Biological Control, 45*, 404–409.

Klein, M. G. (1990). Efficacy against soil-inhabiting insect pests. In R. Gaugler & H. K. Kaya (Eds.), *Entomopathogenic Nematodes in Biological Control* (pp. 195–214). CRC Press.

Koch, M. S., Ward, J. M., Levine, S. L., Baum, G. A., Vicini, J. L., & Hammond, B. G. (2015). The food and environmental safety of *Bt* crops. *Frontiers in Plant Science, 6*, 283–336.

Koppenhöfer, A. M., & Fuzy, E. M. (2008). Early timing and new combinations to increase the efficacy of neonicotinoid–entomopathogenic nematode (*Rhabditida: Heterorhabditidae*) combinations against white grubs (*Coleoptera: Scarabaeidae*). *Pest Management Science, 64*, 725–735. https://doi.org/10.1002/ps.1550 (accessed on 2nd January 2026).

Koppenhöfer, A. M., Choo, H. Y., Kaya, H. K., Lee, D. W., & Gelernter, W. D. (1999). Increased field and greenhouse efficacy with a combination of entomopathogenic nematode and *Bacillus thuringiensis* against scarab grubs. *Biological Control, 14*, 37–44. https://doi.org/10.1006/bcon.1998.0663 (accessed on 2nd January 2026).

Koppenhöfer, A. M., Kostromytska, O. S., McGraw, B. A., & Ebssa, L. (2015). Entomopathogenic nematodes in turfgrass: Ecology and management of important insect pests in North America. In R. Campos-Herrera (Ed.), *Nematode Pathogenesis of Insect and Other Pests* (pp. 309–327). Springer International Publishing. https://doi.org/10.1007/978-3-319-18266-7_12 (accessed on 2nd January 2026).

Lacey, L. A., & Georgis, R. (2012). Entomopathogenic nematodes for control of insect pests above and below ground with comments on commercial production. *Journal of Nematology, 44*, 218–225.

Li, E., Qin, J., Feng, H., Li, J., Li, X., Nyamwasa, I., Cao, Y., Ruan, W., Li, K., & Yin, J. (2021). Immune-related genes of the larval *Holotrichia parallela* in response to entomopathogenic nematodes *Heterorhabditis beicherriana* LF. *BMC Genomics, 22*, 192. https://doi.org/10.1186/s12864-021-07506-4 (accessed on 2nd January 2026).

Li, Z., Alves, S. B., Roberts, D. W., Fan, M., Delalibera, I., Tang, J., Lopes, R. B., Faria, M., & Rangel, D. (2010). Biological control of insects in Brazil and China: History, current programs and reasons for their successes using entomopathogenic fungi. *Biocontrol Science and Technology, 20*, 117–136. https://www.researchgate.net/publication/281766568_Mass_Production_of_Entomopathogenic_Fungi_State_of_the_Art (accessed on 2nd January 2026).

Lomer, C. J., Bateman, R. P., & Johnson, D. L. (2001). Biological control of locust and grasshopper. *Annual Review of Entomology, 46*, 667–702.

Lord, J. C. (2005). From Metchnikoff to Monsanto and beyond: The path of microbial control. *Journal of Invertebrate Pathology, 89*(1), 19–29. https://doi.org/10.1016/j.jip.2005.04.006 (accessed on 2nd January 2026).

Lozano-Gutiérrez, J., & España-Luna, M. P. (2008). Pathogenicity of *Beauveria bassiana* (Deuteromycotina: Hyphomycetes) against the white grub *Laniifera cyclades* (Lepidoptera: Pyralidae) under field and greenhouse conditions. *Florida Entomologist, 91*, 664–668.

Luthy, P., Cordier, J., & Fischer, H. (1982). *Bacillus thuringiensis* as a bacterial insecticide: Basic considerations and application. In E. Kurstack (Ed.), *Microbial and Viral Pesticides* (pp. 35–74). Marcel Dekker.

Marrone, P. G. (2009). Barriers to adoption of biological control agents and biological pesticides. In *Integrated Pest Management* (pp. 163–178). Cambridge University Press.

Martineau, B. (2001). *First Fruit: The Creation of the FlavSavr Tomato and the Birth of Biotech Foods* (p. 269). McGraw-Hill.

McIntosh, A. H., Rice, W. C., & Ignoffo, C. M. (1987). Genotypic variants in wild type populations of baculovirus. In K. Maramorosch (Ed.), *Biotechnology in Invertebrate Pathology & Cell Culture* (pp. 305–325). Academic Press.

Menn, J. J., & Hall, F. R. (2001). Biopesticides—Present status and future prospects. In J. J. Menn & F. R. Hall (Eds.), *Methods in Biotechnology, Vol. 5: Biopesticides Use and Delivery* (pp. 1–9). Humana Press.

Meyer, S. L. F., Huettel, R. N., & Sayre, R. M. (1990). Isolation of fungi from *Heterodera glycines* and *in vitro* bioassays for their antagonism to eggs. *Journal of Nematology, 22*(4), 532–537.

Meyer, S. L. F., Johnson, G., Dimock, M., Fahey, J. W., & Huettel, R. N. (1997). Field efficacy of *Verticillium lecanii*, sex pheromone, and pheromone analogs as potential management agents for soybean cyst nematode. *Journal of Nematology, 29*(3), 282–288.

Milner, J. R. (2000). Current status of *Metarhizium* as a mycoinsecticide in Australia. *Biocontrol News and Information, 21*(2), 47–50.

Mishra, J., Tewari, S., Singh, S., & Arora, N. K. (2015). Biopesticide: Where we stand? In N. K. Arora (Ed.), *Plant Microbes Symbiosis: Applied Facets* (pp. 37–75). Springer.

Moscardi, F., Allen, G. E., & Greene, G. L. (1981). Control of the velvetbean caterpillar by nuclear polyhedrosis virus and insecticides and impact of treatments on the natural incidence of the entomopathogenic fungus *Nomuraea rileyi. Journal of Economic Entomology, 74*, 484–485.

Nagamine, T., Abe, A., Suzuki, T., Dohmae, N., & Matsumoto, S. (2011). Co-expression of four baculovirus proteins, IE1, LEF3, P143, and PP31, elicits a cellular chromatin containing reticulate structure in the nuclei of uninfected cells. *Virology, 417*, 188–195.

Neves, P. M. O. J., & Hirose, E. (2005). *Beauveria bassiana* strains selection for biological control of the coffee berry borer, *Hypothenemus hampei* (Ferrari) (Coleoptera: Scolytidae). *Neotropical Entomology, 34*, 72–82.

Ohkawa, T., Volkman, L. E., & Welch, M. D. (2010). Actin-based motility drives baculovirus transit to the nucleus and cell surface. *Journal of Cell Biology, 190*, 187–195.

Okano, K., Vanarsdall, A. L., Mikhailov, V. S., & Rohrmann, G. F. (2006). Conserved molecular systems of the *Baculoviridae*. *Virology, 344*(1), 77–87. https://doi.org/10.1016/j.virol.2005.09.019 (accessed on 2nd January 2026).

Ortiz-Urquiza, A., & Keyhani, N. O. (2013). Action on the surface: Entomopathogenic fungi versus the insect cuticle. *Insects, 4*, 357–374.

Passarelli, A. L. (2011). Barriers to success: How baculoviruses establish efficient systemic infections. *Virology, 411*, 383–392.

Patel, C. S., Jani, V. B., Parekh, V. B., Darji, V. B., & Vaishnav, P. R. (2009). Genetic diversity and differentiation of *Helicoverpa armigera* nuclear polyhedrosis virus isolates from India. *Phytoparasitica, 37*, 407–413.

Pell, J. K., Eilenberg, J., Hajek, A. E., & Steinkraus, D. C. (2001). Biology, ecology and pest management potential of *Entomophthorales*. In M. T. Butt, C. Jackson, & N. Maga (Eds.), *Fungi as Biocontrol Agents* (pp. 71–115). CAB International.

Pigott, C. R., & Ellar, D. J. (2007). Role of receptors in *Bacillus thuringiensis* crystal toxin activity. *Microbiology and Molecular Biology Reviews, 71*, 255–281.

Prasad, C. S., Singh, R., Prasad, M., & Pal, R. (2011). *Mass Production of Bioagent and Their Uses* (Technical manual, pp. 1–68). SVPUAT.

Quinlan, R. J. (1988). Use of fungi to control insects in glasshouses. In M. N. Burge (Ed.), *Fungi in Biological Control Systems* (pp. 19–85). Manchester University Press.

Ramanujam, B., Rangeshwaran, R., Sivakmar, G., Mohan, M., & Yandigeri, M. S. (2014). Management of insect pests by microorganisms. *Proceedings of the Indian National Science Academy, 80*, 455–471.

Rana, I. S., Kanojiya, A., & Sandhu, S. S. (2008). Mosquito larvicidal potential of fungi isolated from larval mosquito habitats against *Aedes aegypti*. *Journal of Biological Control, 22*, 179–183.

Reardon, R., Podgwaite, J. P., & Zerillo, R. T. (1996). GYPCHECK–the gypsy moth nucleopolyhedrosis virus product. *USDA Forest Service Publication FHTET, 96*, 16.

Roberts, D. W., & Humber, R. A. (1981). Entomogenous fungi. In G. T. Cole & B. Kendrick (Eds.), *Biology of Conidial Fungi* (pp. 201–236). Academic Press.

Rosell, G., Quero, C., & Coll, J. (2008). Botanical biopesticide combination concept—a viable option for pest management in organic farming. *Journal of Pesticide Science, 33*, 103–121.

Sandhu, S. S., & Vikrant, P. (2006). Evaluation of mosquito larvicidal toxins in the extracellular metabolites of two fungal genera *Beauveria* and *Trichoderma*. In G. Bagyanarayana, B. Bhadraiah, & I. K. Kunwar (Eds.), *Emerging Trends in Mycology, Plant Pathology and Microbial Biotechnology*. B. S. Publications.

Sandhu, S. S., Sharma, A. K., Beniwal, V., Goel, G., Batra, P., & Kumar, A. (2012). Myco-biocontrol of insect pests: Factors involved, mechanism, and regulation. *Journal of Pathogens*. https://dx.doi.org/10.1155/2012/126819 (accessed on 2nd January 2026).

Schnepf, E., Crickmore, N., & Van Rie, J. (1998). *Bacillus thuringiensis* and its pesticidal proteins. *Microbiology and Molecular Biology Reviews, 62*, 775–806.

Schuler, T. (1991). *Verticillium lecanii* (Zimmermann) Viegas (Hyphomycetales: Moniliaceae): Geschichte, Systematik, Verbreitung, Biologie und Anwendung im Pflanzenschutz. *Mitteilungen aus der Biologischen Bundesanstalt für Land- und Forstwirtschaft, Berlin-Dahlem, Heft 269*, 154.

Shapiro-Ilan, D. I., Cottrell, T. E., Mizell, R. F., Horton, D. L., & Abdo, Z. (2015). Field suppression of the peach tree borer, *Synanthedon exitiosa*, using *Steinernema carpocapsae*: Effects of irrigation, a sprayable gel, and application method. *Biological Control, 82*, 7–12.

Sharma, R., & Sharma, P. (2021). Fungal entomopathogens: A systematic review. *Egyptian Journal of Biological Pest Control, 31*, 57. https://doi.org/10.1186/s41938-021-00404-7 (accessed on 2nd January 2026).

Sridhar, K. C. (2008). *Development and Evaluation of Diagnostic Tools for Nucleopolyhedroviruses Infecting Major Lepidopteran Pests of Legume Crops in the Semi-Arid Tropics* (Ph.D. Thesis). Department of Biochemistry, Acharya Nagarjuna University.

Srinivasa, M., Jagadeesh Babu, C. S., Anitha, C. N., & Girish, G. (2008). Laboratory evaluation of available commercial formulations of HaNPV against *Helicoverpa armigera* (Hub.). *Journal of Biopesticides, 1*, 138–139.

Sun, X. L., & Peng, H. (2007). Recent advances in biological pest insects by using viruses in China. *Virologica Sinica, 22*, 158–162.

Sung, G. H., Poinar, G. O., & Spatafora, J. W. (2008). The oldest fossil evidence of animal parasitism by fungi supports a Cretaceous diversification of fungal-arthropod symbioses. *Molecular Phylogenetics and Evolution, 49*, 495–502.

Szewczyk, B., Hoyos-Carvajal, L., Paluszek, M., Skrzecz, I., & Lobo de Souza, M. (2006). Baculoviruses: Re-emerging biopesticides. *Biotechnology Advances, 24*, 143–160.

Thakur, R., Jain, N., Pathak, R., & Sandhu, S. S. (2011). Practices in wound healing studies of plants. *Journal of Evidence-Based Complementary & Alternative Medicine*. https://dx.doi.org/10.1155/2011/438056 (accessed on 2nd January 2026).

Upadhyay, V., Rai, D., Rana, M., Mehra, P., & Pandey, A. K. (2014). *Verticillium lecanii* (Zimm.): A potential entomopathogenic fungus. *International Journal of Agriculture, Environment and Biotechnology, 7*(4), 719–727.

Vaek, M., Reynaerts, A., & Hofte, A. (1987). Transgenic plants protected from insects. *Nature, 325*(6125), 33–37.

Van Oers, M. M., & Flak, J. M. (2007). Baculovirus genomics. *Current Drug Targets, 8*, 1051–1068.

Vashisth, S., Chandel, Y. S., & Sharma, P. K. (2013). Entomopathogenic nematodes—A review. *Agricultural Reviews, 34*(3), 163–175.

Wraight, S. P., Jackson, M. A., & de Kock, S. L. (2001). Production, stabilization and formulation of fungal biological agents. In T. M. Butt, C. Jackson, & N. Magan (Eds.), *Fungi as Biocontrol Agents* (pp. 253–287). CABI.

Zhang, C. X., Ma, X. C., & Guo, Z. J. (2005). Comparison of the complete genome sequence between C1 and G4 isolates of the *Helicoverpa armigera* single-nucleocapsid nucleopolyhedroviral. *Virology, 333*, 190–199.

Zimmermann, G. (1984). Pilze zur biologischen Bekämpfung von Blattläusen. *Gärtnerbörse und Gartenwelt, 17*, 406–407.

Index

B

H

I

J

K

T

U

V

For Product Safety Concerns and Information please contact our EU representative GPSR@taylorandfrancis.com Taylor & Francis Verlag GmbH, Kaufingerstraße 24, 80331 München, Germany